Cystic Fibrosis

YOUR PERSONAL HEALTH SERIES

Cystic Fibrosis

EVERYTHING YOU NEED TO KNOW

WAYNE KEPRON, MD, FRCPC

FIREFLY BOOKS

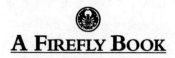

A FIREFLY BOOK

Published by Firefly Books (U.S.) Inc. 2004

First Printing

Publisher Cataloging-in-Publication Data (U.S.)

Kepron, Wayne.
   Cystic fibrosis : everything you need to know / Wayne Kepron.—1st ed.
[196] p. : ill. ; cm. (Your personal health)
Includes index.
Summary: A guide for those diagnosed with cystic fibrosis, and their families.
ISBN 1-55297-740-4 (pbk.)

1. Cystic fibrosis—Popular works. 2. Cystic fibrosis—Treatment—
Popular works. I. Title. II. Series.

616.3/7 21   RC858.C95.K47   2004

Published in the United States in 2004 by
Firefly Books (U.S.) Inc.
P.O. Box 1338, Ellicott Station
Buffalo, New York, USA
14205

Published in Canada in 2003 by Key Porter Books Limited.

Design: Peter Maher
Electronic formatting: Heidy Lawrance Associates

Printed and bound in Canada

Contents

Introduction

The fact that you're reading this book probably means that you are aware of someone who has cystic fibrosis, or that you have cystic fibrosis yourself. The multitude of emotions that come with understanding and accepting the enormity of this diagnosis have likely passed. Rather than addressing these past painful experiences, this book will focus on what can be done now to cope with this illness, and to look forward, with a reasonable degree of optimism, to the future.

The name "cystic fibrosis" came to be used approximately sixty years ago to describe changes found, on autopsy, in young children who had died of a combination of lung infections and problems with digestion and malnutrition. "Cystic" refers to cysts, or small empty spaces, and "fibrosis" refers to associated areas of scarring, found within the pancreas glands of people with this condition.

Cystic fibrosis (CF) was first noted in Northern Europe some four hundred years ago. As the Northern Europeans migrated around the world, the illness was transported to the rest of Europe, North and South America and Australia, and it continues to affect predominantly Caucasian populations on all these continents.

Even though CF was recognized a long time ago, it was only in the late 1930s that the disease was first well described in both Europe and North America. At first this was a devastating diagnosis. Infants, once diagnosed, weren't expected to survive even a year. However, with a better understanding of this illness and continuing improvements in medical and supportive care, the expected survival time has risen dramatically. Average life expectancy has reached 35½ years in most developed countries, and it's now reasonable to expect that, before long, all children diagnosed with cystic fibrosis will survive childhood and reach adulthood. While this is a great achievement in pediatric care, people with CF and their caregivers now must deal with fitting into and managing in an adult world, with all of its added psycho-social issues, as well as all the medical problems of CF that carry over from childhood.

In no other illness has such an organized and focused team approach to treatment been developed. Every person with cystic fibrosis, and his or her family, will come to know a CF clinic doctor, who will most likely be a pediatrician to start, and also a CF clinic nurse and coordinator. As well, patients and families will meet regularly with dietitians, physiotherapists, clinical pharmacists and social workers. As the person gets older, another doctor, most likely a specialist in lung disease, will be added to this team. Other specialists may be asked to assist with complicated problems as they arise. These could include a gastroenterologist (specializing in stomach, bowel and liver problems), an endocrinologist (specializing in endocrine disorders such as diabetes) or perhaps a specialist in adolescent medicine to help in the transition from pediatric-centered care to adult clinic care. Over the past twenty-five years, the contribution of all these individuals has dramatically improved survival rates in people with CF.

Cystic fibrosis is a complex disease, and it may affect more than one organ in the body. This book will explain the basic problem, how the defect in the CF gene affects various organs and how therapy can help deal with the problems. You'll get detailed information about the organs most commonly and most severely affected. Individual chapters discuss how this illness affects the lungs, the pancreas and other digestive organs, and the reproductive system in both the male and the female. Treatments aimed at these specific organs will be dealt with in their own chapters as well.

The problems that people with CF face during childhood are the same problems they encounter during adulthood. However, as they reach adulthood they may also face new problems such as deciding whether to pursue education, choosing a career, coping with sexuality and forming new relationships that extend beyond the family. These concerns will be addressed in the appropriate sections within this book.

New therapies are constantly being devised and introduced into the care plan for people with cystic fibrosis, and those that have been tested in clinical trials and accepted into clinical practice will be reviewed. Current information on lung transplants as it applies to CF is summarized in its own chapter, and the current status and future prospects of gene therapy will also be reviewed. It's not within the scope of this book, however, to look at therapies still under investigation, or those that are thought to have promise but haven't been adequately assessed yet. For the same reason, there will be no discussion of the basic science research being conducted so actively in many laboratories today.

Cystic fibrosis is an illness that touches all family members and may come to involve a significant portion of their lives. With their care and support comes the hope that even more people with CF will soon be able to reach middle age and beyond.

ONE

What Is Cystic Fibrosis?

C ystic fibrosis is a genetic disorder, which means that it's determined by the genes a person inherits from his or her parents. As many as 60 percent of people with CF are diagnosed within the first one to two years of life and this number rises to 85 percent by five years of age. However, up to 10 to 15 percent will be over the age of eighteen when the diagnosis of CF is finally established. We don't know why the time when symptoms first appear varies so greatly. It may be due in part to the large number of gene defects that are now known to exist in different people (see Chapter 2 for more details). CF most commonly appears as recurrent and, very often, persistent lung infections. Another significant problem that shows up is the failure of normal growth and development in early childhood, the result of chronic poor nutrition in people with untreated CF. These individuals aren't able to digest and absorb food normally, due to the way CF affects the pancreas and the digestive tract. Many other organ systems may be involved as well, and these will all be discussed in more detail in the chapters that follow.

Incidence of CF in different countries	
Country	Number of live births resulting in one baby with CF
Ireland	2,000
France	3,000
North America	3,500
Sweden	8,000
Finland	40,000
Asia	90,000

How Common Is This Disease?

Cystic fibrosis occurs at different rates in different races and ethnic populations. It most commonly affects Caucasians, with one newborn in every 2,500 live births being ultimately diagnosed with CF. By comparison, the African American population will have only one child in every 17,000 births diagnosed with this disease, and in most Asian groups only one in every 90,000 births results in cystic fibrosis. Males appear to be slightly more likely to get CF than females. At the present time, approximately 3,000 people in Canada and 30,000 people in the U.S.A. have cystic fibrosis.

How Is the Disorder Inherited?

To have CF, a child must receive a defective CF gene from both mother and father. The parents may have CF, or may be "carriers" of the disease. In Chapter 2 we'll look at what genes are and how they come to be passed from parent to child.

What Can Be Expected for People with CF?

The average lifespan of people with CF has increased steadily since this disorder was first recognized. In 2002, a child born with CF could be expected to live somewhere between thirty-five and forty years. Every clinic now reports that patients are surviving into their forties and occasionally even into their fifties. With improvements in medical care, the development of lung transplantation and perhaps with gene therapy in the future, people with CF will continue to live longer and may someday even approach normal lifespans.

What Are the Symptoms and Signs of Cystic Fibrosis?

Tara was born to healthy parents and had a normal five-year-old sister. Although slightly small at birth she appeared otherwise normal. Her mother described her as having a voracious appetite from birth. As she was switched from breast milk to infant formulas, her usually loose stools became decidedly bulky, foul-smelling and pale in color. Her mother noticed that the stools tended to float in the toilet, and that Tara's stomach always appeared to be distended. Tara's doctor, noting that she didn't gain weight as expected and didn't appear to grow in length, ordered a sweat chloride test. The results were positive. A second positive sweat chloride test confirmed the diagnosis of CF, and further genetic testing showed that Tara did indeed possess the most common CF gene defect.

Tara was referred to a CF clinic for further follow-up. After an assessment by the clinic physician and a dietitian, she was started on pancreatic enzymes. The little girl rapidly gained weight, her stools became normal in color and consistency and her abdominal distention disappeared.

When cystic fibrosis appears early in infancy, as in Tara's case, complaints related to the bowels, nutrition or failure to grow are the most common indications. Later on in childhood, breathing difficulties become much more prominent. Unexplained coughing or episodes of pneumonia that don't appear to respond

Signs and symptoms that may warrant testing for CF

- nasal polyps in an infant or child
- prolonged jaundice in an infant
- pain in nasal or facial sinuses
- recurrent wheezing episodes
- persistent cough with yellow/green sputum
- frequent productive cough
- coughing up blood
- recurrent "pneumonias"
- meconium ileus (bowel obstruction) in an infant
- bulky, foul-smelling stools
- failure to grow (referred to as "failure to thrive")
- rectal prolapse (protrusion)
- male infertility

or clear completely with therapy become much more common. When people aren't diagnosed until later in life, respiratory symptoms appear to be the main problem that prompts testing for cystic fibrosis.

How Is the Diagnosis Established?

A doctor will often suspect CF in an infant or a small child showing poor growth, a failure to grow (referred to as "failure to thrive"), chronic chest symptoms or chronic bowel problems. Once CF is suspected, a diagnosis can be made using an easy and very accurate procedure called the sweat chloride test. If the level of chloride in the sweat is elevated, a diagnosis of CF becomes a very strong possibility. Most doctors accept a diagnosis of CF if the sweat chloride test is positive, *and* if two of the following are also present:

Sweat chloride test

The sweat chloride test remains the standard test for the diagnosis of cystic fibrosis today. The test is easy to perform, can be done at any age, is painless and inexpensive and produces a result within a few hours.

The sweat in people with CF contains a high concentration of chloride ions, which makes it taste saltier. This concentration can be easily and accurately measured. A small amount of a chemical called pilocarpine is placed on the skin of the forearm, back or leg. A weak electrical current is then applied to this area for five to ten minutes. (The current is rarely felt by the person.) The combination of electrical current and pilocarpine causes the sweat glands to produce an increased flow of sweat, which can be collected by a filter paper during the next thirty to sixty minutes and can then be analyzed for chloride ion content. Most physicians require that at least two positive tests be obtained before a diagnosis of CF is made.

Some other conditions are also associated with elevated sweat chloride. Most of these, though, can easily be diagnosed by other means and are not often confused with cystic fibrosis.

- persisting gastrointestinal symptoms
- persisting chest symptoms
- a family history of cystic fibrosis

Genotyping, or CF Gene Detection

Genetics laboratories can now detect and identify the CF gene in the majority of those affected, through a process referred to as genotyping. Because testing is expensive and involved, it's currently not used as a screening procedure, but only to confirm a diagnosis of CF following a positive sweat chloride test. Also, most laboratories can only identify somewhat less than 10 percent of the total number of gene defects (over eight hundred) which have so far been described. Although most defects would be identified in North America by these screening procedures, some diagnoses could be missed simply because of this limitation. Fortunately, the sweat chloride test detects all CF patients, and therefore remains the screening test of choice in all clinics.

Common Early Symptoms and Signs of Cystic Fibrosis

Meconium Ileus

Meconium is a substance that fills the bowel or intestines at birth. It's a normal secretion of the intestines, and is composed largely of mucus. It's usually expelled when the infant first feeds, and in a normal infant it produces no symptoms. In the CF-affected infant, though, the meconium is very thick and can't be easily expelled. Instead, it lodges within the bowel, usually where the small intestine joins the large intestine, and may cause a bowel obstruction (ileus). A baby with this condition will have trouble feeding and may appear to be suffering from colicky pain. If this condition is not recognized, the baby may develop vomiting as well. Up to 10 percent of newborn infants who are ultimately diagnosed with CF have meconium ileus. Occasionally this plug of meconium can be gently washed out with special enemas. Sometimes, however, an operation may be required to remove the plug, and in more severe cases a small portion of the bowel may also be removed, because it's often damaged by the obstruction.

Failure to Thrive

Infants with CF may initially appear to have a voracious appetite and yet fail to grow and gain weight normally. This "failure to thrive" is apparent within the first six months of life and is evident to some degree in about 70 percent of newly diagnosed CF patients. Failure to thrive occurs because the normal digestive process is interfered with: the pancreas fails to function normally and to provide the enzymes necessary to digest foods. The baby will pass bulky, greasy, pale and very foul-smelling stools, because the fats in the diet aren't fully digested and are therefore not absorbed by the intestine. This is a form of malnutrition.

Incidence of early warnings of CF

Warning	Percent affected
acute or persistent respiratory symptoms	50.5%
failure to thrive	43%
abnormal stools	35%
meconium ileus	19%
family history of CF	17%
rectal prolapse	3.5%
positive result in neonatal screening	2.0%
nasal polyps	2.0%

Rectal Prolapse

Approximately 10 percent of untreated CF infants develop a bulging of the lining of the large bowel that protrudes out through the rectum. Although it is not known exactly why this *prolapse* of the bowel occurs, it may be the result of passing fatty, bulky stools through the large intestine. A rectal prolapse does not appear to be a major problem; it will usually clear up once enzyme therapy is started to aid digestion, and normal bowel movements are restored.

Respiratory Symptoms

Cough and Sputum

The age at which breathing symptoms appear can vary greatly. Most often, respiratory symptoms show up as a stubborn cough described as being very loose or "rattly." This cough tends to persist despite attempts at treatment. Young children may have persistent wheezing or recurrent pneumonia. Older children may produce sputum, and it is not uncommon for the sputum to be yellow to green in color. As lung disease progresses, coughing and the production of yellowish or green sputum will become a constant feature, occurring on a daily basis.

Coughing Up Blood

Coughing up blood (*hemoptysis*) tends to be more common in older patients, and often occurs without warning. While this may be associated with a worsening of the lung infection, it may also occur without any apparent cause. Fortunately, these episodes usually stop on their own and don't produce any serious side effects. However, in rare cases they persist, and special procedures may be needed to control the bleeding.

Clubbing of the Fingers and Toes

As lung problems develop, it's quite common to see the ends of the fingers and toes enlarge and become rounded, with the fingernails becoming much more curved than normal. This is called *clubbing*, and it appears to parallel the progression of the lung disease in CF. It's not clear why this happens. As the disease progresses, the tips of the fingers and toes, as well as the lips, may also appear bluish in color, due to falling levels of oxygen in the blood.

Nose and Sinus Symptoms

Polyps develop within the nasal cavities of up to 10 percent of people with CF. These polyps are simply swellings of the normal lining of the nasal cavity. It's not clear exactly why this happens, but in some instances the polyps interfere significantly with breathing through the nose. Because the polyps may also obstruct the sinuses around the nose, symptoms of sinusitis (swollen sinuses) are common too. People with sinus symptoms usually complain of pain about the face, or headaches.

Symptoms in the New Adult CF Patient

As many as 10 percent of all people with CF aren't diagnosed until after the age of eighteen. In this group, lung problems are the usual tip-off. These individuals will experience persistent

Warnings of adult-onset CF

Warning	Percent affected
recurrent respiratory infections	92%
screening with positive family history	24%
gastrointestinal complaints	8%
infertility (usually males)	4%

cough with yellow-green sputum, signs that can't be explained by the usual lung diseases seen in young adults. Some individuals are infertile. Very often, when such symptoms can't be explained, doctors carry out a sweat chloride test.

TWO

The CF Gene— What Went Wrong?

G enes are quite extraordinary. They control what we look like and how every small part of our bodies functions. Genes determine whether we have black hair or red hair, whether we become tall or short, and in addition they control all of our organ functioning from day to day. There are a vast number of genes in the body, which allow each of us to be unique and different from other individuals. Genes are passed from parents to children and then on to their children, so that family characteristics are passed from generation to generation. A defect in a gene may likewise be passed from parent to child; this is probably most striking in those who suffer from hemophilia or, as we shall see, in cystic fibrosis. When a disease is transmitted by an abnormal gene, it's called a genetic disorder, or a genetic disease.

Genes and Chromosomes

Genes are components of chromosomes, which are microscopic structures that carry hereditary information within each cell of our bodies. Each of our cells contains twenty-three pairs of chromosomes, each pair perfectly matched, with one of the pair coming from the mother and the other from the father. Chromosomes can be identified by their appearance under a microscope. Once identified, they're assigned numbers 1 through 22. The remaining pair of chromosomes defines whether we are male or female, so these two are usually called the sex chromosomes.

Chromosomes are long strand-like structures made up of many genes linked end to end. Each individual gene is always found on the same chromosome, and is always in the same position on that chromosome. Each gene is unique in structure and always performs the same function, throughout the life of the individual. For example, one gene is responsible for controlling the production of insulin within the pancreas, and that's the only thing it does. In the same way, each hormone and each enzyme in the body is controlled by its own unique gene, which has no other function. Scientists have been able to identify many genes, and to recognize where they reside on different chromosomes.

The Structure of a Gene

A gene itself is made up of many small molecules linked end to end to form long strands of deoxyribonucleic acid—or as it's more commonly called, DNA. DNA is formed by two strands of these molecules wound around each other in a spiral fashion and held together by "crossbridges." The small building-blocks of molecules are called *nucleotides*. There are only four different nucleotides, and they're arranged in sequences, like a code. The particular pattern made by a specific sequence defines the message that the gene sends out to the cell to produce a certain structure or function.

The cystic fibrosis gene alone consists of up to a quarter of a million nucleotides. With only four different nucleotides to work from, it's easy to see how complex the combinations and sequences must be to form the 250,000 positions on the DNA chain of the CF gene.

We still don't know exactly how many different genes there are on the twenty-three pairs of chromosomes, but there may be as many as a hundred thousand. They must obviously differ to some degree, or we would all come out looking the same. Some genes, though, are *always* the same (or very nearly the same) from person to person. We know this because, for example, insulin has the same structure from one person to another; therefore the insulin must be produced by a gene that is also identical from one person to another. With such a huge number of possible combinations of nucleotides within a gene, some variation in the normal function of a gene may be possible— a slight variation in a gene makes one person's hair black and another's blond. However, other variations in gene structure are distinctly abnormal, and when these variations occur, they can result in significant illness.

Several gene alterations have been described that explain certain genetic disorders, and many more will likely be described in the near future. But what is the gene defect in cystic fibrosis, and how does it produce this disease?

What Causes CF—a Gene Gone Wrong

In 1989, Dr. Lap-Chee Tsui and collaborators described the gene associated with cystic fibrosis, and localized it to the long arm of chromosome number 7. This particular gene defect was identified as the most common defect present in North Americans with CF, being found in about 70 percent of them. It's called the delta F508 defect—the delta ("d") standing for deletion, the "F" for the particular building-block that is missing (phenylalanine), and 508 for the position in the DNA strand where the defect was found. Since this initial discovery, over 800 other gene defects producing CF have been identified, among the 250,000 building-blocks forming the CF gene. These hundreds of other defects account for the remaining 30 percent of CF patients. What's amazing about this particular defect is how the loss of a very small molecule, which can't even be seen by the most sophisticated scientific equipment, can result in such a serious and as yet incurable disease. Having this knowledge gives us hope that, some time in the near future, scientists may find a way to correct this defect and, as a result, find a cure for CF (see Chapter 10 for more on gene therapy for CF). As this gene is the site of the genetic defect resulting in CF, it has become known as the "CF gene." This can be confusing, as the gene is *normal* in people unaffected by CF. When CF is being discussed, as in this book, the term "CF gene" usually refers to the abnormal gene.

What Is the Result of Having the Abnormal Gene?
The CF gene is responsible for producing a channel, or pump, that is normally inserted into the surface of cells lining the various ducts in the liver, pancreas, testicles, sweat glands, intestines and airways of the lungs. This channel is called the *cystic fibrosis transmembrane regulator*, or *CFTR* (sometimes the CF gene is called the CFTR gene, since its only function is to control production of the CFTR). As with the term "CF gene," the inclusion of "CF" in the name only reflects the importance of this channel in the mechanism of CF. Once produced and inserted into the cells, the CFTR acts as a gate mechanism that controls how much water is allowed to pass across the cell membrane. This passage of water in turn controls the thickness of the secretions or mucus within the ducts of various organs, or within the airways of the lungs. (This control is largely achieved by the cell pumping chloride ions back and forth across the cell membrane, through the CFTR channel.) In cystic fibrosis, an abnormal CF gene results in not enough

The cystic fibrosis transmembrane regulator (CFTR)

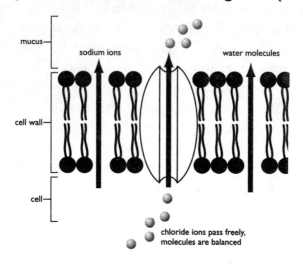

mucus—

sodium ions

water molecules

cell wall—

cell—

chloride ions pass freely,
molecules are balanced

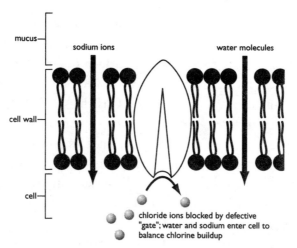

mucus—

sodium ions

water molecules

cell wall—

cell—

chloride ions blocked by defective
"gate"; water and sodium enter cell to
balance chlorine buildup

A normal CFTR moves chloride ions out of the cell and into the mucous layer within the ducts and airways. Sodium and water are shifted through separate channels, in response to the movement of the chloride. Above, when the CFTR functions correctly, there is a balance between the chloride ions and the sodium. Below, an abnormal CFTR cannot move chloride out of the cell. Sodium ions move into the cell, to balance the excess chloride. Water then follows, to keep the sodium concentration at normal levels within the cell. Because this water has come from the mucous layer, the mucus is reduced in volume, and has a much thicker consistency.

of the CFTR protein being produced and inserted into the cell surface. As a result, the production of normal mucus within the ducts or airways breaks down, and instead a very thick mucus is produced. The ducts or airways become plugged by this mucus, and these tiny structures are damaged. This in turn causes further damage to the various organs, resulting in the characteristic symptoms and physical signs of CF. The specific effects on various organs will be discussed in the following chapters.

Cystic Fibrosis and Heredity

Remember that we inherit our characteristics from both parents. Only one chromosome from each of the twenty-three pairs is present in either the egg or the sperm. When the egg and sperm unite, the two sets of chromosomes once again pair up, the mother's chromosome 1 with the father's chromosome 1, and so on. As each cell then grows and divides, it always reproduces the twenty-three pairs of chromosomes.

If only one of the chromosome 7 pair carries an abnormal CF gene, no disorder will occur in the person carrying this defect. However, this person will be a *carrier* of the CF gene. But if the person inherits an abnormal CF gene from *each* parent, then both chromosomes will carry the abnormal gene, and the person will develop CF. Both chromosomes *must* carry an abnormal CF gene before CF will occur. The CF gene abnormalities inherited from the two parents do not have to be identical for CF to occur. For example, CF will result even if the very common delta F508 gene defect from one parent is paired with a less common defect from the other parent.

Can We Predict Cystic Fibrosis?

If you have CF, and you decide to have children, the CF defect will be passed on to your child. Since CF only occurs when *both* parents pass on a defective gene, your partner can be tested to see if he or she is a carrier with a defective CF gene. Since most labs can't screen for all CF gene abnormalities, we can't be completely sure that an apparently unaffected partner doesn't carry some abnormal CF gene. However, as most common defects can be tested for, we can be reasonably confident in predicting the chance that a child will be born with CF.

Who Should Be Tested?

Most people with CF today have already been tested (*genotyped*) to determine which particular gene defect they have. This information is used by geneticists and CF foundations to help define patterns of disease in people with different types of gene defects. Occasionally it is also used to predict whether mild or severe symptoms are likely to develop in a child, to help guide parents in their treatment and plans. It's a good idea for everyone with CF to be genotyped to identify the specific gene defect.

Sometimes, individuals without CF are tested to see if they carry the abnormal CF gene—perhaps when a person with CF and a non-CF partner consider having a child, or when two individuals who appear unaffected but have strong family histories of CF are considering having a family. Since CF carriers are symptom-free, only testing can show whether or not a single defective gene is carried by one or both partners.

Calculating the Risk of CF

A child can be born with CF only if both parents are carriers of a defective CF gene, or if one parent has CF and the other parent is a carrier of a defective CF gene. One of the two chromosomes in each parent is passed on to the child, but the chromosome that's passed is determined purely by chance. Where both parents are carriers, the child could inherit one normal

Heredity patterns in cystic fibrosis

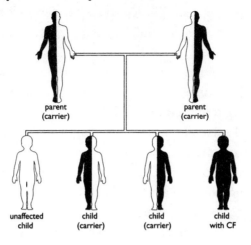

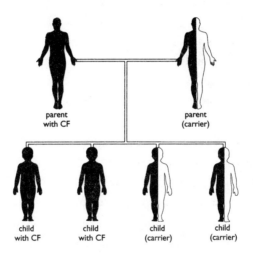

chromosome from each parent, and be unaffected; both chromosomes could be abnormal and the child would have cystic fibrosis; or the child could inherit an abnormal gene from one parent and a normal one from the other parent, and would then appear unaffected but would be a carrier of this abnormal gene. Thus, if two carrier parents have children, on average:

- 25 percent of their children will have CF;
- 50 percent of their children will be carriers of the CF gene;
- 25 percent of their children will be unaffected.

It is important to remember that the chromosome pairings are completely by chance. If a child born to this couple has CF, it *does not* mean that their next child will be unaffected, or will be a carrier. Each child born to this couple will have a one-in-four chance of having CF as well.

What if one parent has CF and the partner is a carrier? Then we can predict that, on average:

- 50 percent of their children will have CF;
- 50 percent of their children will be carriers of the CF gene;
- no children will be unaffected.

Similarly, if one parent has CF and the other parent doesn't carry a CF gene, all their children will be symptom-free carriers of the CF gene.

We've seen how someone may carry the abnormal CF gene without knowing it. The number of undetected carriers of an abnormal CF gene may be as high as 3 percent of the population, so it's not unlikely for two such affected individuals to meet, marry and have children—and one child in four will have CF. For the foreseeable future we'll continue to see CF children being born without prior warning because the parents appear unaffected. At present, we don't screen for carriers in the general population, because the tests are expensive and technically difficult to perform in large numbers. If simple, inexpensive screening tests become available, earlier detection of people at risk for having a CF child may be possible. For now, though, genetic screening is only recommended to those with a strong history of CF in their immediate families.

Are There Other Ways of Looking at the Risks?

When someone with CF develops a relationship with another person, he or she may not know whether that person carries the abnormal CF gene. Since not all abnormal CF genes can be detected by all laboratories, the risk always remains, however small it may be. It's possible to make a rough calculation of the risk, based on the following family conditions of the person in question.

Both mother and father have a brother or sister with CF	1 in 9
Both mother and father have a nephew or niece with CF	1 in 16
Either mother or father has a brother or sister with CF	1 in 150
Either mother or father has a nephew or niece with CF	1 in 200
No history of CF in either family	1 in 2,500

Bill and Sylvie were newly married and considering starting a family. Sylvie knew of a cousin in another city who had cystic fibrosis. Concerned that their child could be born with the disorder, they went to their family doctor for guidance. She arranged for them to see a CF clinic physician, who explained to the couple that, because of Sylvie's family history of cystic fibrosis, they had a greater chance of having a baby born with CF than a couple with no family history of the illness. With the cooperation of Sylvie's cousin and her CF doctor, it was determined through testing that her cousin had the most common gene defect responsible for CF. In order to relieve both Sylvie and Bill's anxieties, genetic testing was arranged to see if either of them carried the CF gene. This testing didn't detect any of the common gene defects in either Bill or Sylvie, and it was highly unlikely they were both carrying one of the rare gene defects that current procedures don't test for. As a result, Sylvie and Bill were told that there was little chance they would ever have a child with CF, and that they should go ahead with planning a family.

Other Testing Options for CF

Prenatal Testing

Sometimes, parents would like to know if a pregnancy will result in a CF child being born—if, for example, the parents both have a strong family history of CF and haven't been tested themselves. A CF mother with a partner who is a carrier has a 50 percent chance of having a child with CF; these parents may want to know whether the child is in fact going to be born with CF.

Two procedures are available for prenatal testing. The first is *chorionic villus sampling*, and can be done as early as ten to thirteen weeks into the pregnancy. A small catheter, or tube, is inserted into the mother's cervix and then into the uterus. A few cells are removed from the placenta by gentle suction and are tested for the abnormal CF gene.

The second procedure is *amniocentesis*. This involves inserting a needle through the wall of the mother's abdomen and into the uterus. Amniotic fluid, which contains cells shed by the fetus, is withdrawn. These cells are likewise examined for the abnormal CF gene.

Can Any Other Type of Screening be Done?

As we've seen, because of the cost and complexity of the tests, screening is only carried out when there's a strong family history of CF. But since the abnormal CF gene can be present in people who appear unaffected, scientists are trying to find other screening methods to diagnose CF very early in children—perhaps even in newborns—who don't have a strong family history of the disease. The theory is that early diagnosis and treatment, before symptoms of CF become apparent, may reduce or delay the development of symptoms, and may even help these children have longer lives. Attempts to detect CF in newborns are called *neonatal screening.*

How Does Neonatal Screening Work?

Neonatal screening is testing done on babies as early as three to five days old. The screening involves a very simple blood test called the *immunoreactive trypsin test,* or IRT. The test can be done using the same sample of blood that is now routinely taken from each infant shortly after birth to screen for other inherited diseases, such as phenylketonuria (PKU). The IRT detects increased levels of trypsin and trypsinogen, which are enzymes released from the pancreas. In the newborn infant with CF, the effect of the disease on the pancreas results in small amounts of these enzymes being released into the bloodstream. The enzymes can be detected by this very sensitive test. However, the test doesn't provide a true CF diagnosis, because small levels of these enzymes may be present in some unaffected babies. For this reason, a follow-up test must be done when the infant is between two and eight weeks old. This is a major drawback to this type of testing, as some of the infants will have a normal follow-up test, and the parents will have been worrying needlessly in the interim. If the follow-up test is positive, a second type of test will be have to be performed—usually the sweat chloride test discussed previously. This test is deferred until the baby is five to eight weeks of age.

Why Bother with Neonatal Screening?

There are two arguments put forward in favor of screening newborns. As noted above, some people argue that starting therapy at a very early age might favorably alter the course of the illness, reducing its severity and the need for hospitalizations as well as prolonging life expectancy. Several countries have carried out these tests, but the results have varied widely from country to country. Because there hasn't been a definitive answer as to whether or not early detection alters the course of CF in a useful way, most countries haven't adopted any form of neonatal screening for CF. The National Institutes of Health in the United States recommends that widespread neonatal testing not be implemented at the present time, pending further studies to see whether this kind of testing is a reasonable approach to detecting and diagnosing CF.

However, as testing procedures become easier, or as new test procedures are developed, some form of more widespread screening may become available in the future.

THREE

CF and the Respiratory System

To understand cystic fibrosis, we first have to understand the respiratory system, which in humans begins with the nose. The nasal openings connect with the nasal passages, which in turn lead to the throat, and to the larynx (voicebox). The larynx contains the vocal cords, and it's at the level of the vocal cords that the opening to the lungs actually occurs.

The Nasal Passages

The nasal passages have several functions. The passages are lined by a special layer of cells that secrete a thin lining of mucus, which acts to trap particles and bacteria that might be inhaled with each breath. This is a major role of the nasal passages: by acting as a filter system, they provide a defense against these bacteria or particles, which might cause injury if inhaled into the lungs. Along the walls of the nasal passages are folds of tissue called *nasal turbinates*; they warm the inhaled air as the air passes through the nose. At the same time, water is added by the turbinates, to humidify the air before it enters the lungs. Very dry air might damage the delicate lining membranes of the lungs, if it were inhaled over a long period of time.

Surrounding the nasal passages and lying within the bones of the skull are several air-filled spaces (cavities) called sinuses. No one knows exactly why sinuses exist, as they don't seem to have any specific function (except maybe to make our skulls lighter!) These sinuses—the frontal, maxillary and ethmoid sinuses—are lined by the same mucus-secreting membrane that lines the nasal passages. Mucus is produced within these sinuses on a daily basis, and drains into the nasal passages through narrow passageways. From the nasal passages the mucus drains down to the back of the throat, and is then swallowed, without our even realizing that this occurs. Occasionally, disease involves the sinuses (usually infections) or the nasal passages (usually polyps), and both these conditions are very common in people who have CF.

Sinus Disease

Fourteen-year-old Julio had complained of occasional nasal stuffiness and nasal discharge over several years. He had been diagnosed with CF at the age of three, but his symptoms were generally quite mild and were usually relieved by the occasional use of a decongestant. Apart from using enzymes with meals and daily vitamin supplements, he used no other medication and had few problems related to his CF.

One summer Julio's nasal stuffiness returned and persisted despite his usual treatment. When he went to the clinic, doctors found a nasal polyp in his right nostril and marked swelling of the membranes lining his nasal passages. They recommended decongestant tablets and a local nasal spray, which gave Julio relief for a little while. One day, though, he felt a dull, aching pain in his right cheekbone and he complained of feeling feverish.

An X-ray showed fluid in the sinuses in both Julio's cheekbones. In fact, his right sinus was completely filled with fluid.

His doctor prescribed an antibiotic, which controlled the infection that was producing this episode of acute sinusitis. In the following months, Julio went through similar episodes. Although they were controlled with decongestants and antibiotics, the condition had now become chronic and doctors suspected that he had developed a persisting infection in the sinus cavity.

Julio was sent to an ear, nose and throat specialist, who suggested that the sinus should be drained. After explaining the procedure to Julio and his parents, the surgeon created a small opening between the nasal cavity and the sinus. This allowed the fluid to drain, and relieved the pressure within the sinus cavity. As soon as this pressure was relieved, Julio's pain disappeared instantly, and he experienced no further episodes.

For some unknown reason, sinuses may not develop normally in CF. Up to one-third of all people with CF don't have a well-developed frontal sinus. Sinus disease may occur in any of the sinuses, and up to 10 percent of children and up to 25 percent of adolescents and adults experience symptoms. After adolescence the incidence of sinus disease seems to decline, for reasons that aren't clear.

The same processes that affect the lungs, the pancreas and other duct systems in someone with CF also involve the nose and nasal passages. The mucus that is normally produced within the sinuses is much stickier and thicker than the mucus found in an unaffected person. This thickened mucus can block the ducts that normally drain the sinuses into the nasal cavities. Once an obstruction occurs within these ducts, the sinus becomes much more susceptible to infections from different bacteria. Localized infection and the inflammation that infection produces within the sinuses are called sinusitis. When this occurs suddenly, as the result of a new infection, it's called acute sinusitis. When the infection is prolonged, with daily symptoms over several weeks or months, it's called chronic sinusitis.

Symptoms of sinus disease

- facial pain
- jaw or tooth pain
- forehead pain
- nasal discharge

- facial swelling
- fever
- post-nasal drip

Once an infection develops, the increased inflammation causes an increased production of secretions, and the sinus fills up entirely with fluid. Since the fluid can't drain properly through the blocked ducts, pressure builds up, and this pressure produces the characteristic symptom of sinusitis—severe pain in the area immediately above the affected sinus. Pain felt above the eyes is most commonly due to involvement of the frontal sinus, and pain in either the right or left side of the face, just below the eye, most commonly involves the maxillary sinuses. When the maxillary sinus is involved, there may also be pain in the upper jaw or along the teeth on the affected side. When an active infection is present, the part of the face over the involved sinus will often feel tender if you press the bone firmly with your finger. Occasionally, people with CF may notice increased discharge from the nose as the yellow or yellow-green secretions drain from the various infected sinus cavities. These secretions may even drain backward and be felt in the back of the mouth and throat. This is referred to as post-nasal drip.

Often, when X-rays of the skull or sinuses are taken, the sinuses appear to be filled with fluid and yet no symptoms are present. In these instances, no treatment is necessary or warranted.

Treatment of Sinus Disease

Antibiotics. When an infection is severe and is producing significant symptoms, antibiotics may be required. The infection is most commonly caused by pseudomonas bacteria or, occasionally, by hemophilus bacteria. Oral antibiotics are usually prescribed, and the antibiotic chosen depends on the specific organism causing the infection.

Decongestants. These medications are generally applied directly to the nasal passages, through the use of a spray preparation. Decongestants shrink the lining membrane of the nose and open the drainage duct from the sinuses. This helps to promote drainage from the affected sinus cavity, which in turn will relieve the pressure symptoms of pain.

Drainage of the sinus cavity. Occasionally, when symptoms are severe or recurrent and can't be controlled by antibiotics and decongestants, drainage of an infected sinus may be considered. This requires referral to an ear, nose and throat specialist. Drainage usually involves piercing the wall of the affected sinus and introducing a small, telescope-like instrument called a *nasoscope* into the sinus cavity. The nasoscope allows the sinus cavity to be inspected for severity of disease, and allows for irrigation of the cavity with sterile solutions. The nasoscope can also drain secretions, which will reduce the pressure in the cavity and relieve the pain. Although these procedures may provide very effective and very quick relief, symptoms frequently recur and repeated drainage procedures may be necessary.

If symptoms persist despite this therapy, other drainage procedures may be considered. One such procedure involves inserting a small plastic catheter into the sinus cavity and leaving it in place, taped to the cheek, to wash the sinuses out three to four times a day. Antibiotics can then be inserted directly into the infected sinus to help eradicate the bacteria causing the infection. As well, sterile salt solutions may be used to wash out thickened mucus and inflammatory fluids, and to help relieve pain from the pressure. Some lung transplant centers advocate this type of treatment prior to performing a transplant in a CF patient.

Finally, as a last resort for persistent sinusitis, it's sometimes possible to create a permanent opening from the sinus directly into the nasal passage. This operation, which is done by a surgeon, requires a general anesthetic and is usually only performed for very severe and persistent sinus symptoms.

Nasal Polyps

Nasal polyps are the second most commonly occurring nasal passage problem encountered by people with CF. A polyp is simply a localized swelling of the lining membrane of the nasal passage. As this swelling develops, it causes the membrane to bulge outward. When sufficiently enlarged, the swelling appears as a cyst-like, rounded structure bulging into the nasal cavity. If polyps become very large, or if multiple polyps develop, they can cause a significant degree of obstruction within the nose.

Nasal polyps are detected in anywhere from 10 percent to 33 percent of all persons with CF, and are most commonly found in children with CF between the ages of five and fourteen. For some unknown reason, polyps often disappear by early adulthood. Since nasal polyps are very rare in children without CF, finding a polyp or polyps in a child should always raise the question of CF, if it hasn't already been diagnosed.

Symptoms of nasal polyps

- polyps visible in nasal opening
- loss of sense of smell
- halitosis (bad breath)
- nosebleed
- nasal obstruction
- snoring, mouth-breathing
- nasal discharge

Polyps obstruct the nasal passages and prevent normal airflow through the nose. The most common symptom is an inability to breath adequately through the nose. The obstruction may also cause snoring at night and may interfere with normal sleep. Other symptoms may be a loss of the sense of smell, nosebleeds, halitosis (bad breath) and, very commonly, nasal discharge.

Treatment of Nasal Polyps
Decongestants and antihistamines. When symptoms aren't too severe, nasal decongestants or antihistamines may be enough to keep the symptoms under control and to allow the individual to breathe relatively comfortably through the nose. Success with this treatment, and with all medical therapy, varies. When there is some inflammation due to ongoing infection in the nose, these medications may provide some relief.

Steroid preparations. Similarly, spray preparations containing corticosteroids may be applied directly to the polyps to try to reduce any swelling in the membranes or lining of the nasal cavity. This may be particularly effective if an allergy such as hay fever (also thought to be more common in people with CF) is present. Corticosteroid sprays, like decongestants and antihistamines, may not always be effective.

Surgery. When symptoms of obstruction become severe and interfere with breathing, surgery is the most effective form of treatment for polyps. The procedure, called a *polypectomy*, is a relatively simple operation. It involves cutting the polyp off at the base, and removing it from the nose. Unfortunately, in most people who have symptoms secondary to polyps, this procedure doesn't always produce permanent results. Up to 90 percent of patients undergoing polypectomy will have the

polyps recur, and they may have to undergo repeat polypec-
tomies to continue to control their symptoms.

Lung Disease in Cystic Fibrosis

Debbie required her first admission to hospital for CF at the
age of four. She awoke one morning with a very harsh cough
and a temperature above 103°F (almost 40°C). She was taken
to the CF clinic, where a chest X-ray showed pneumonia in
the left lung and she was admitted to the hospital for treatment. A throat swab and a specimen of her sputum grew a
bacteria called staphylococcus, which is commonly found in
children with CF. Her pediatric CF doctor prescribed an intravenous antibiotic and within thirty-six hours Debbie's temperature was down to normal. At the same time as she started
on antibiotics, Debbie was seen by a physiotherapist who
started her on a program of chest physiotherapy three times a
day during her hospital stay. Several days later, when Debbie's
condition had improved, the physiotherapist met with her
parents to review home physiotherapy for Debbie. When she
was ready to be discharged, the physiotherapist also set up
an outpatient plan to be sure that her mother and father had
a regular review of techniques for their daughter's care. The
physiotherapist instructed her parents in proper chest physiotherapy, and encouraged them to participate in Debbie's physiotherapy during the remainder of her hospital stay.

In an unaffected person, the small cells lining the airways of the
lungs continuously produce a layer of mucus that coats the entire
surface of the airways. This layer forms a protective barrier to
trap any particles or bacteria that enter the lungs during normal
breathing. The mucous layer is normally swept out of the lung
by the action of very small, hair-like projections called *cilia*, which
stick out of the surface of the airway cells. The cilia beat con-

tinuously, and this beating motion sweeps the mucus and any trapped particles or bacteria out of the lung and into the throat. The mucus is then swallowed without us being aware that this has happened, as is the mucus from the sinuses.

In most people with CF, the lung appears to be structurally normal at the time of birth, but changes begin to occur at a very early age. As we saw in the previous chapter, the thickness of the mucous layer is controlled by the CFTR protein in the surface of the cells lining the airways, but people with CF have defective CFTR in their cell walls, so that the cells are unable to control the flow of chloride ions and water. As a result of this abnormal flow of water, the mucus is much thicker and stickier than normal, and much more difficult to move out of the airways. This thickened layer of mucus also prevents the cilia from beating properly. The cilia can't move this abnormal layer upward and out of the lungs, as they would normally, and the very thick and sticky fluid tends to accumulate in all the small airways of the lungs.

Now, the bacteria that occasionally enter the lungs during normal breathing and stick to this layer can't be expelled normally, and become trapped in the small airways. Once this occurs, infections may develop; normal mucus produced in the airway appears to inhibit the growth of any bacteria that penetrate the lungs, but the abnormal mucus produced in the CF airway seems to have lost this ability. The inflammation produced by the multiplying bacteria may then injure the walls of the small airways, causing even more obstruction, which leads to even more inflammation, which results in even more obstruction—and the cycle continues.

Initially, and often within the first year of life, the changes of obstruction and inflammation involve the *bronchioles* (very small airways) of the lungs. When this is severe enough to cause coughing and wheezing, it's called *bronchiolitis*. Eventually this inflammatory process may produce so much damage that the airways are partially destroyed and balloon outward to form small cyst-like areas. This condition is called *bronchiectasis*, and the development of bronchiectasis is considered the hallmark change in the lungs in CF; once it occurs, the changes are always permanent, because the airways aren't able to heal themselves even when antibiotics are used to combat the infections. The bronchiectatic areas are prone to developing even more infections, and it's very likely that these areas are the starting point for the occasional acute pneumonia that people with CF may experience.

This cycle of inflammation and infection may begin in early childhood, and it's a chronic ongoing process once it's established. Its major effect is the production of much more mucus than the airways would normally produce, and this excessive mucus is the cause of the excessive sputum production that eventually develops in most people with CF.

Lung Infections

The reason for the shortened life expectancy of people with CF is respiratory failure, the result of destruction of the lungs by infections. Active infection and inflammation in their lungs may be detected as early as the first year of life. Infections are detected by sending a specimen of sputum to a bacteriology laboratory, where bacteria can be grown (*cultured*), identified as to type and tested to see which antibiotics will kill them. Several different bacteria may be cultured in the sputum of persons with CF at different times of their lives. Some of the commoner bacteria are as follows.

Staphylococcus

This is one of the first organisms that appear when we culture sputum from infants and children with CF. Luckily, this bacterium is sensitive to treatment with a wide variety of antibiotics. Eventually the staphylococci seem to be replaced in older people with CF by pseudomonas bacteria (see below), but they may occasionally be found along with the pseudomonas.

Hemophilus

This bacterium also appears to be found mostly in babies and children, and tends not to be cultured from sputum once pseudomonas appears. Hemophilus seems to be a very common organism, and often shows up in patients with ear, nose and throat problems as well as lung problems in the younger age groups. Like staphylococcus, it is sensitive to a wide variety of antibiotics.

Pseudomonas

Pseudomonas aeruginosa is the commonest and most important infection in adults with CF. Pseudomonas may start appearing in early childhood; as people with CF age, it shows up more and more, and it's found in up to 80 percent of all adults with CF. Pseudomonas occurs widely throughout nature and we're exposed to it throughout virtually all daily activities. Probably the most common place to find pseudomonas is in hospitals, where this organism can be cultured from virtually every room, every sink and almost all hospital equipment. Because it's so commonly found in nature, infection most likely comes from the environment and is probably less likely to come from an already infected person.

When found in the environment and cultured in the laboratory, the pseudomonas colonies are described as being "rough," or *nonmucoid*, which refers to their physical appearance on the medium or substance used to grow the bacteria. After infecting a patient, the pseudomonas can transform to produce a thick, slimy coating which produces a very smooth, shiny colony when grown on the culture medium. This is called the *mucoid* or "smooth" form of pseudomonas. Both the non-mucoid and the mucoid forms appear in sputum cultures from CF patients.

Pseudomonas is a difficult organism to deal with. Once established in the lungs, it will stick to the surface of the cells lining the airways and, as a general rule, can never be wiped out. The slimy layer formed by this bacterium probably protects it from the person's normal defense mechanisms, such as white blood cells, and also likely hinders antibiotics when they attack it. Pseudomonas also produces a variety of enzymes and toxins which, when released during each acute infection, will cause more local tissue damage and further bronchiectasis. With treatment we can control the symptoms and hope to limit tissue damage, but treatment will *never* completely get rid of the pseudomonas organisms in the airway.

Burkholderia Cepacia—A Special Case

Burkholderia cepacia (cepacia to most people) became a CF-related problem only in the 1980s. When it first appeared in people with CF, it caused major deterioration in lung function, and many of these people didn't live as long as they'd been expected to. Not surprisingly, this made the CF community very apprehensive, with people assuming that infections from this bacterium would automatically lead to an early death. Over time, though, it became clear that only about 20 percent of those infected with cepacia experience rapid lung deterioration. The remaining 80 percent appear to have the same decline in lung function as people infected by the other commonly seen bacteria.

Originally we thought cepacia was related to pseudomonas, so it was called *pseudomonas cepacia*. Now it's considered to be a separate and distinct bacterium. Cepacia can be found all through our environment; in fact, it turns out that this organism is what causes onion rot, and spoilage in many other vegetables as well. It can be useful, though; it's widely used in agriculture and is sprayed on vegetable crops to control fungal growth. Cepacia is even used to clean up environmental spills of various toxic agents. Because of its widespread use, some people are worried that we're all becoming more and more exposed to cepacia, which could seriously affect the CF community.

In most CF clinics, only 3 to 10 percent of people are ever infected with cepacia. Some clinics have had higher percentages, but lately, with the use of strict control measures (see below), these clinics have had fewer cases. By comparison, some 60 to 80 percent of people are infected with pseudomonas.

As with all other organisms that infect people with CF, once cepacia appears in the sputum it's very hard—if not impossible—to get rid of it completely. The infection can take several different courses.

- Some people are infected yet show no change in symptoms or lung function. These people are considered cepacia "carriers." They can go on for a long time, perhaps forever, with no symptoms, despite the fact that the organism is present in their sputum.
- Other people deteriorate slowly over months or years, with intermittent fevers, weight loss and repeated hospital stays when their CF flares up.
- Some mildly infected people suddenly experience a severe deterioration in lung function. In the past this was known as "cepacia syndrome," but fortunately, it now affects only about 20 percent of people infected with cepacia.

Why Should We Be So Concerned about Cepacia?
Cepacia is a particular problem because it's very easily transmitted from one person with CF to another. One person even

carried this organism from North America to a clinic in the United Kingdom, and caused several people in that clinic to be infected as well. Once cepacia's ability to spread from person to person was recognized, clinics throughout both North America and Europe adopted strict precautions to try to control its transmission from patient to patient and, of course, from clinic to clinic.

These control measures are necessary because cepacia isn't very sensitive to the usual antibiotics used to treat the various infections that people with CF are prone to. Some people need multiple antibiotics to control cepacia infections, and even they may not be effective.

Family members, friends and other social contacts who don't have CF don't seem to become infected with cepacia. However, once a family member with CF becomes infected with cepacia, any other family member with CF will eventually become infected as well. Following the control measures may delay the spread of cepacia to others with CF, or perhaps even prevent it altogether.

Cepacia and Lung Transplantation

Several transplant centers have reported that people infected with cepacia don't appear to do as well as non-cepacia patients following lung transplants. In fact, some centers simply won't do transplants on cepacia-infected patients. Other centers will consider the cepacia-infected patient for transplantation if the cepacia organisms seem sensitive to any antibiotic. Bear in mind, however, that chances for a successful operation are definitely not as good for someone who has cepacia. Whether lung transplants are offered in this case depends on the individual lung transplant program involved, and may vary from region to region, in both Canada and the United States.

> ## Measures to avoid transmission/ acquisition of Burkholderia cepacia
>
> Once cepacia is found in the sputum of someone with CF, the doctor must report this to the person as soon as possible, explaining that this organism is easily passed between people with CF, and that the precautions listed below should be followed consistently.
>
> - Avoid close contact with other people with CF in confined spaces such as physiotherapy rooms, hospital rooms, exercise rooms, etc.
> - Don't share physiotherapy or respiratory therapy equipment such as nebulizers, aerochambers, PEP masks or flutter valves, or metered-dose inhalers such as bronchodilators.
> - Avoid sharing personal items such as toothbrushes, cups, plates, eating utensils, etc.
> - Always cover your mouth when coughing or sneezing.
> - Go to the special cepacia CF clinic, or go to the regular CF clinic at the end of clinic hours.
> - Avoid going to CF-sponsored events such as annual meetings or retreats.
> - Avoid close personal contact, such as kissing or other intimate acts, with people who have CF but do not have cepacia.
>
> When admitted to hospital, people with cepacia should be given single rooms, or specific rooms assigned by the infection control staff.

Symptoms and Signs of Lung Disease in People with CF

Coughing and Sputum

The earliest and eventually most distressing symptom that people with CF lung disease complain about is the development of a cough. Coughing is a natural defense mechanism of the body, and it happens with most forms of lung disease. Probably the most common cause of cough in cystic fibrosis is the production of huge amounts of very thick, sticky sputum in the lower airways. As this sputum accumulates, the body's natural tendency is to try to cough it out, to keep the airways clear for breathing. Other things can cause coughing, though. Remember that there's always some degree of inflammation in the airways, the result of the ongoing bacterial infections. This inflammation is in itself an irritant to the airways, and the lungs no doubt also produce a cough to try to get rid of this irritation.

As the infection and resulting inflammation slowly progress, the production of sputum increases as well. The person will cough more, and the coughing episodes may become more severe. Eventually the person may be coughing every day, and may even be awakened at night by coughing spells.

Wheezing

Wheezing occurs when the airways become filled with the heavy sputum. It may also happen when the airways become constricted or develop spasm from the inflammation caused by the ongoing infection.

Shortness of Breath

Shortness of breath, or "air hunger," is the feeling of not being able to get enough air into the lungs with each breath. Initially you may experience this with heavy exertion or exercise, even though it hasn't been a problem previously. Again, one major reason is the inflamed and obstructed airways—a breath of air simply can't get down into the lungs. Another reason is that the lung tissue itself becomes damaged by the ongoing infection and loses its ability to take up oxygen. When the blood oxygen level falls, your muscles can't work efficiently, because they need oxygen for energy production. The brain, sensing this lack of oxygen, tries to compensate by having the lungs increase both the rate of breathing and the size of each breath. This means added work for your chest muscles as they try to move more air in and out of the damaged and less efficient lungs. Not surprisingly, you end up feeling hungry for air, or short of breath.

Blood in the Sputum (Hemoptysis)

If you have CF, you should probably expect to have at least one episode of coughing up bright red blood, and it may happen more than once. Unfortunately, hemoptysis is unpredictable and often occurs suddenly, with absolutely no warning. The bleeding originates in the damaged areas of the lung, where bronchiectasis has developed and where blood vessels become dilated, when one of these dilated blood vessels ruptures. Infections seem to increase the chance of hemoptysis, but you can have absolutely no other symptoms, and no signs of active infection, and still have blood in your sputum. Fortunately, the hemoptysis usually stops on its own, without requiring any drastic measures to control it. (See also Complications of Lung Disease—Hemoptysis, later in this chapter.)

Lung Sounds

If you listen through a stethoscope to the lungs of a person with cystic fibrosis, you may hear "crackles"—sounds coming from the areas affected by bronchiectasis. They are probably produced by the increased and very sticky sputum that accumulates in these spots. It may also be possible to detect wheezing in some people, which likely represents areas of obstruction within the lungs, either from secretions or from spasms in the airways resulting from the inflammation.

Clubbing

As mentioned in Chapter 1, people with CF, especially those with advanced or severe lung disease, often have swollen and enlarged fingertips and tips of the toes. It's not clear exactly what causes this clubbing, but it appears to develop as the lungs become more infected. Clubbing also tends to develop as the level of oxygen falls in the bloodstream. It should be noted that clubbing may be found in individuals with other lung diseases, and may even be found in some people with chronic bowel disorders.

Monitoring Lung Condition

A person with CF spends a good deal of time visiting the health-care team and undergoing a variety of tests on a routine basis.

Pulmonary Function Testing (PFT)

The most important routine test is pulmonary function testing. Eventually, the obstruction of the airways will lead to measurable changes in lung function, which can be readily detected by PFT. The test best suited to monitor change in lung function measures the amount of air that can be pushed out of the lung in the first second of a forceful exhaled breath. This test is called the FEV_1 (pronounced F-E-V-one. FEV stands for "forced expiration volume"). Although many other measurements of lung function are recorded during PFT, the FEV_1 is the test most often used to assess the extent and severity of disease involving the lungs and airways, and to follow the changes in lung function as lung disease progresses.

Arterial Blood Gas Test (ABG)

The arterial blood gas test is used to measure the levels of oxygen and carbon dioxide in the bloodstream, which can give us a very good picture of how the lungs are working. That's because with every inhalation our lungs take in oxygen, which the body needs to function and produce energy, and with each exhalation they expel carbon dioxide. (Carbon dioxide, a natural byproduct of breathing, becomes harmful if not constantly removed from our bodies.) As the lungs deteriorate, they can't take in as much oxygen or get rid of as much carbon dioxide, so monitoring the levels of those gases is an excellent way to track changes in lung function over long periods of time.

Arterial blood gas test

ABG shows the pressure (P), or level, of oxygen (O_2) and carbon dioxide (CO_2) dissolved in the blood. This is measured in millimeters of mercury (mmHg). The level of acidity—the pH of the blood—is also reported.

Factor	Normal range
PO_2 (oxygen)	80–100 mmHg
PCO_2 (carbon dioxide)	35–45 mmHg
pH (acidity)	7.35–7.45

As lung disease becomes more severe, the blood oxygen level will start to fall and usually, at the same time, the carbon dioxide level will start to rise.

The arterial blood gas test is done by drawing blood from an artery (usually at the wrist). This involves a small needle prick in the skin, which is no worse than the usual needle poke for drawing blood from the arm for all the other tests that people with cystic fibrosis have to undergo. Getting blood from an artery is tricky, so with children a capillary gas test, sometimes referred to as "cap gas," is used; a tiny pinprick is made on the end of the child's finger, and just a small drop of blood is taken. This test doesn't yield quite as accurate measurements as an ABG, but it's certainly easier on the child.

When a blood gas test shows that a person's oxygen level has fallen below a certain point, it may be time to start continuous home oxygen therapy. When the carbon dioxide level starts to rise above normal, a lung transplant may be looked at as a treatment option (see Chapter 10, "Lung Transplantation and Gene Therapy").

Oximetry

The level of oxygen in the blood can be estimated using a *pulse oximeter*. When clipped on a finger or earlobe, this little device uses a sensor to estimate the level of oxygen through the skin. An oximeter can't measure blood oxygen precisely, but it's an easy way to follow trends in oxygen levels, and may be used each time a person visits the CF clinic. Unfortunately, a similar device to measure carbon dioxide levels in an outpatient setting isn't yet available.

Exercise Oximetry

Often, a physiotherapist will help determine the degree of physical impairment resulting from lung disease through what's known as a six-minute walk test. The patient and the physiotherapist simply walk over a measured course for six minutes, and the distance the patient is able to cover is recorded. During the test, the physiotherapist measures the oxygen saturation of the body by using a pulse oximeter. Because the test is straightforward and can be easily repeated, it provides a way of tracking how the person's ability to function changes from month to month or year to year. If oxygen levels fall consistently below 90 percent, this will usually alert the CF team to the fact that lung disease is progressing and that new treatment options should be looked at.

Chest X-rays

Chest X-rays can be used as part of a routine examination, or as a follow-up examination, because they give a permanent and easily reviewed record of changes that occur in the course of lung disease. While a chest X-ray can't accurately show just how much lung disease is present, it can detect the progression of the disease, and X-rays have the advantage of being a very simple procedure. One thing an X-ray can show is bronchiectasis first developing in the upper lobes of the lungs—a unique feature of CF—as opposed to in the lower lobes, where other lung conditions (such as emphysema) start.

Computerized Tomography (CT) Scans of the Chest
These scans are a variation of the chest X-ray examination, and they give us similar permanent images of the lung. The CT, however, can provide much more accurate information about lung changes, and can document these changes very precisely over time. The problem is that this test takes more time than an ordinary chest X-ray, and it's also much more expensive. Also, the patient must lie absolutely motionless for twenty seconds while the scan is done.

Occasionally the doctors wish to look at the blood vessels of the lung in greater detail. This may be done by repeating the scan after a dye has been injected into a vein in the arm.

The CT scan is safe and doesn't cause any discomfort to the patient. Most clinics don't use CT scans routinely, but they will order them when they want a more accurate picture of the lungs. A CT exam will be performed routinely as part of any assessment undertaken for a lung transplant.

Complications of Lung Disease

Pneumothorax
Pneumothorax literally means "air in the chest," and about one in five people with CF will experience it at some point. Because it's associated with more severe lung disease, pneumothorax appears more often in adults, and relatively infrequently in children. The pneumothorax occurs when a small hole develops in the lung, usually in the cyst-like areas that occur with CF lung disease, and allows part of each breath to leak out of the lung and into the chest cavity. The air that escapes then surrounds the lung and causes it to partially collapse.

James was a twenty-two-year-old university student who went to the adult CF clinic regularly. Morning and evening physiotherapy helped control his cough and sputum production. One day, while attending classes, he experienced a sudden dull, aching pain on the right side of his chest. As soon as the pain started, he also felt short of breath, even though he was sitting still. He quickly went to the hospital emergency room, where a chest X-ray showed that he had a pneumothorax. James was admitted to the hospital for observation and given oxygen for twenty-four hours by nasal catheter, but the pneumothorax persisted. Doctors then inserted a small plastic tube between his ribs and into his right chest cavity. Once the air had been completely drained from the pneumothorax, the tube was taken out. James was discharged and he returned to his classes three days later.

Two weeks following his discharge from hospital, James experienced the same symptoms again, except this time he felt even more short of breath. Another chest X-ray confirmed that his pneumothorax had recurred and was larger than the previous one. James went back into the hospital. This time, a thoracic surgeon was called in to treat him. The surgeon made a small incision on the right side of James's chest, and examined the exposed lung for abnormalities such as cysts that might have ruptured to produce the pneumothorax. No obvious rupture or cyst was present, so the surgeon gently abraded the lung with a cotton swab to make it stick to the chest wall and prevent it from collapsing again. Several days later, James was able to go home. He continues to be seen regularly in the adult CF clinic, and he hasn't had another recurrence of his pneumothorax.

Symptoms of a Pneumothorax

Very often the person notices sudden, strong chest discomfort or pain on the same side as the pneumothorax. At the same time, he or she may suddenly feel extremely short of breath, and this shortness of breath may continue as long as the lung is partially collapsed. When symptoms persist or become really distressing, the most common treatment is to drain the air out of the chest cavity and re-expand the lung as quickly as possible.

Treatment of a Pneumothorax

Treatment depends on the size of the pneumothorax, which can vary from person to person, and the intensity of the symptoms. Treatment options might include:

- admitting the person to hospital for observation only
- draining the pneumothorax with the insertion of a chest tube
- operating to correct any lung defects and to prevent further recurrences of the pneumothorax

Most people will be admitted to hospital for monitoring, and to make sure that the pneumothorax doesn't get worse. Someone who is only mildly short of breath may be admitted and treated with nasal oxygen until the hole causing the air leak seals itself, which it will almost always do. Giving the person additional oxygen to breathe seems to help the pneumothorax heal faster. This approach should only be taken, though, if the pneumothorax is small or if the person feels only very mildly short of breath. The major drawback of this approach is that up to 25 percent of people with this problem will have their pneumothorax recur within a year.

When symptoms of pain or shortness of breath are more severe, doctors may decide to remove the air from the lung cavity. They do this by inserting a plastic tube between the ribs and into the chest cavity, but not into the lung itself. Gentle suction is then applied to the tube, which sucks the air out of the chest cavity and makes the lung expand. The tube is left in place until the hole in the lung seals over and no more air escapes into the chest cavity. This usually takes about twenty-four to forty-eight hours. Once the lung has expanded, the tube can be removed and the person can go home.

Unfortunately, a pneumothorax is very likely to recur, even after successful drainage. For this reason, it's often deemed advisable to carry out a further procedure called a *pleurodesis*, to try to prevent recurrences. The goal is to make the lung fuse or stick to the chest wall so that it can't collapse again. There are basically two ways to achieve this. The type of pleurodesis used depends largely on whether the person is considered a candidate for a lung transplant in the future.

Chemical Pleurodesis

This is the most effective method of pleurodesis. Once the collapsed lung has been re-expanded, a substance—usually talc—is flushed through the chest tube directly into the chest cavity. The substance acts as an irritant and causes an inflammation of the lining of the lung, and also of the lining of the chest wall itself. The inflammation causes the lung to stick to the chest wall. This method is usually very successful in preventing further incidents of pneumothorax. There are drawbacks, though, to this procedure. The irritation and inflammation may cause a great deal of discomfort, which lasts for about twenty-four to forty-eight hours. Also, the fusion of the lung to the chest wall makes it virtually impossible to remove that lung in the future, essentially preventing the person from ever having a lung transplant.

Abrasion Pleurodesis

This is the preferred method of preventing pneumothorax in people who might later be considered for a lung transplant. With the patient anesthetized, a surgeon makes a small incision in the armpit area. Through this incision, the surgeon can directly inspect the top part of the lung, where most pneumothoraxes originate. If the hole causing the pneumothorax can be identified, the surgeon can close it with either sutures or staples. Then the surface of the exposed lung is gently abraded with a cotton swab to cause a mild inflammation, which fuses the lung to the chest wall. This type of pleurodesis appears effective in preventing further pneumothoraxes from occurring, yet it doesn't produce as dense adhesions as chemical pleurodesis. Most transplant surgeons will do a lung transplant in a patient who has had an abrasion-type pleurodesis.

Hemoptysis

Carrie was diagnosed as having cystic fibrosis when she was ten, and she was started on twice-daily physiotherapy to help clear her thick yellow sputum. With regular physiotherapy and an occasional course of antibiotics to control acute flare-ups of her symptoms, she required no hospital admissions until she was thirteen years of age, when she suddenly coughed up several tablespoons of bright red blood. Carrie and her parents were extremely upset, and immediately contacted their CF coordinator and physician. Carrie told them that she had noted a slight increase in cough and slightly more sputum production for two days before the bleeding. A chest X-ray showed no significant changes. Carrie was put on an antibiotic to treat this apparent flare-up of symptoms and was allowed to go home, but was encouraged to call the CF coordinator if there was further bleeding, to discuss how it might be managed. When another episode did occur, there was less blood than the first time. Carrie telephoned the clinic on her own, and she was reassured that coughing up blood is a common complication in CF. She was also reassured that most episodes of bleeding stop without treatment.

As mentioned earlier, most people with CF experience hemoptysis, or coughing up blood, when blood vessels in damaged areas of the lung rupture. The blood eventually finds its way into an airway and is coughed up. Treatment usually involves admitting the person to hospital, particularly if it's the first episode and if the amount of blood seems large. Because we think hemoptysis develops as a result of infection, most doctors prescribe an antibiotic as part of the treatment. Physiotherapy is usually put on hold until the bleeding stops.

Most episodes of hemoptysis stop on their own, and involve less than one ounce (20–30cc) of blood. Sometimes, though, the person coughs up more than eight ounces (250cc) of blood. This is called massive hemoptysis. When this occurs, or when hemoptysis persists unchanged over several days, more aggressive treatment may be used.

Bronchoscopy

The first step in dealing with a massive hemoptysis is to examine the airways of the lungs, to determine which of the lobes is actively bleeding. This is done with a telescope-like instrument called a bronchoscope. For children, a general anesthetic may be necessary. For adults, the mouth, tongue and throat are "frozen" with a local anesthetic spray so the patient won't feel the bronchoscope as it is passed into the lung. Unless the patient is critically ill, an intravenous sedative will be administered before this, to relax the person as much as possible; with this type of preparation, up to 70 percent of people do not even remember the procedure being done.

It may take five to ten minutes to inspect all the airways. The only aftereffects are an occasional sore throat or mild cough, and possible hoarseness from irritation of the vocal cords by the bronchoscope. All symptoms usually go away within twenty-four hours.

Bronchial Artery Embolism

Once the doctor has figured out where the bleeding is coming from, a radiologist may try to plug the blood vessel that seems to be responsible for the bleeding. This procedure, called an embolization, is technically quite involved and does cause the patient some discomfort. The skin above a vein in the upper thigh and groin area is frozen with an injection of a local anesthetic. The vein is then punctured with a large needle, and a catheter is introduced through the needle into the vein, and advanced to the heart and into the blood vessels of the lungs. The patient must lie very still and try not to cough while dye is injected to outline the blood vessels on a screen. It may require several injections of dye to identify the blood vessel suspected of bleeding, and each injection causes some discomfort, as the dye produces a hot flush. Once the suspected blood vessel is identified, small beads of inert material or small coils of wire are injected to plug it up. This stops the blood flow through the vessel, which in turn stops the bleeding and the coughing up of blood.

While this procedure can work very well, there are so many abnormal blood vessels in a damaged lung that bleeding may happen again, weeks or even months after an apparently successful treatment.

Lobectomy

When bleeding continues despite all attempts to stop it, it may be time to consider surgically removing the part of the diseased lung that's bleeding. This is a very serious decision, because it usually means removing a whole lobe of the lung—as much as 20 to 25 percent of the total lung tissue. This may not be possible if the person already has reduced lung capacity or lung function. On the other hand, such surgery can be lifesaving for someone who has massive and uncontrolled hemoptysis. Luckily, this drastic measure is rarely necessary.

Atelectasis

If an airway becomes completely plugged with secretions, the lung tissue beyond the plugged-up part will collapse, because all the air in that part of the lung is absorbed by the lung tissue. This is called *atelectasis*. If a large section of lung collapses, symptoms may get worse, especially shortness of breath. Treatment involves removing the plug of secretions from the airway by increasing physiotherapy to the affected part of the lung, and encouraging drainage from that area. When physiotherapy can't dislodge the mucous plug, it may have to be removed in a more direct way, by passing a bronchoscope into the lung. The bronchoscope is used to dislodge the secretions and to suck them out of the airway.

Pneumonia

The damaged areas of the lung are very prone to developing pneumonia, which happens when bacteria multiply unchecked and invade the lung tissue. The result is increased cough, increased sputum production, shortness of breath and either chills or fever. When symptoms aren't too severe, these episodes may be controlled by oral antibiotics. If the pneumonia gets worse, though, the person may be admitted to hospital and given intravenous antibiotics. Once the symptoms are under control, the person can often complete the treatment at home through a home IV program, which allows him or her to administer the antibiotics personally.

Respiratory Failure

As lung disease progresses, a time will come when the lung can't take in enough oxygen for normal daily activities, or can't remove the carbon dioxide produced by the body's daily functioning. When this happens temporarily, it's called acute respiratory failure. When lung disease gets worse, chronic respiratory failure can develop.

Acute Respiratory Failure

Occasionally, with a pneumothorax, pneumonia or atelectasis, someone with moderately severe lung disease develops acute respiratory failure. Oxygen levels fall while carbon dioxide levels rise, and the person must be hospitalized. Once the cause for the acute respiratory failure is treated and lung function is restored, the carbon dioxide and oxygen levels will return to normal, as long as no permanent damage to the lung has occurred.

Chronic Respiratory Failure

Eventually the lung disease in everyone with CF progresses to the point where the lung can't remove carbon dioxide from the body adequately, and the level of carbon dioxide in the blood rises slowly. This is called chronic respiratory failure, and it's another indication that a lung transplant should be considered.

Right Heart Failure

The blood vessels passing through the parts of the lung damaged by CF will also become damaged by the infections in these areas. This causes increased pressure in the main blood vessels in the lungs, and this in turn puts a strain on the right ventricle of the heart, which pumps the blood through the lungs. The result of this strain is to slow the blood flow from the veins of the body into and through the right ventricle, resulting in increased back pressure in all the veins that drain into the heart. The increased pressure causes blood fluids to leak out of the veins and into the body tissues; this is most noticeable in the lower extremities, and appears as swelling (edema) of the feet and ankles. Edema may be controlled for a period of time by using diuretics (water pills) to remove fluids from the body.

Treatment of Lung Disease

Physiotherapy
The main treatment for people with CF is always chest physiotherapy, which is started once the symptoms of cough and sputum production develop. The major goal is to prevent mucus from blocking the airways and to remove it efficiently and effectively from the body. See Chapter 8 for information on the various kinds of physiotherapy.

Treatment of Infections
A major part of the treatment of CF-related lung disease revolves around the use of various kinds of antibiotics, chosen according to the type of bacteria found in the person's sputum. Antibiotics are often given by mouth but, depending on the circumstances, may also be administered intravenously or by inhalation (see Chapter 8).

Bronchodilators
While physiotherapy clears mucous obstructions, it can't clear the obstructions caused by spasms in the airways, resulting from infection and subsequent inflammation. Bronchodilators are substances, usually inhaled, that relax the airways that are in spasm. They can be inhaled from small metered-dose inhalers that are easy to carry around in a pocket or purse.

Bronchodilators may also be administered from *nebulizers,* which produce a very fine spray of medication.

Corticosteroids
People with CF sometimes develop wheezing from airflow obstruction, similar to asthma. In fact, when they are tested in the PFT laboratory, the irritability in their airways looks much like asthma. Because corticosteroids help people with asthma, they're used to treat people with CF as well.

Corticosteroids can be inhaled just as bronchodilators are inhaled. In fact, they generally work best in those people with airway obstruction who get good results with a bronchodilator. For this group, adding an inhaled corticosteroid may well improve their lung function and maintain this improvement over a long period of time. Corticosteroids should be taken regularly at the same time every day, at a dose recommended by your CF physician.

An oral form of corticosteroid (usually prednisone) may also be used. This medication is usually taken for only a short time—ten days or less—and seems to be most useful for acute flare-ups of lung symptoms. In these cases, prednisone seems to encourage a speedier recovery.

Inhaled DNase

Deoxyribonuclease, or DNase, is an enzyme that breaks down the protein DNA found in sputum. The breakdown process partially liquefies the sputum and makes it much easier for a person to cough it out. We'll look at this treatment more closely in Chapter 10.

F O U R

CF *and the* Gastrointestinal System

The gastrointestinal system, or digestive system, is made up of the organs responsible for the digestion of our daily diet. The process of digestion involves breaking down the food we eat into smaller components, which can then be absorbed by the intestines. These components are carbohydrates (basically sugars for energy production), fats (largely for energy production) and proteins (for building and maintaining normal muscle and other body tissues). The gastrointestinal tract absorbs other important elements such as calcium, which we need for building and maintaining healthy bone, as well as vitamins, required for normal body function.

The important parts of the gastrointestinal system are the stomach, the pancreas, the liver and the small and large intestines. The digestive process begins at the mouth, where chewing breaks down food and mixes in enzymes produced by our saliva glands. Enzymes are small proteins that break foods down for absorption by the small intestine. The saliva from the salivary glands contains a lipase (an enzyme that starts to digest fats) and an amylase (an enzyme that digests carbohydrates).

When we swallow, the partially prepared food passes from the mouth to the stomach through a long narrow tube called the esophagus. The stomach continues the digestive process by adding acid and an enzyme called pepsin, to begin the digestion of proteins. When the food is thoroughly mixed with acid and enzymes, it's then passed into the small intestine. There, additional enzymes are added from the pancreas, the important ones being the proteases, which further break down protein, and more lipases, which continue to digest fats. At the same time, bile salts from the liver are added to this mixture. Bile salts aid in absorbing the digested food, particularly fats, as they pass along the intestine. Digested food that's either not completely broken down or not absorbed then passes into the large intestine. Here, excess water is removed and any remaining food content gets expelled as stools through the rectum.

Most people with CF develop some problem with some part of the digestive system. Where does this process go wrong, and what changes can be expected as a result?

The Esophagus

Normally, the acid produced by the stomach is prevented from backing up into the esophagus by a small valve at the lower end of the esophagus (the *gastroesophageal sphincter*). Occasionally this valve doesn't work well, and acid is allowed to *reflux*, or back up, into the lower esophagus. We don't know why the valve doesn't always work, but the reflux of acidic stomach content produces a burning sensation or burning pain behind the breastbone. This symptom, called *gastroesophageal reflux disease* (GERD) or, more commonly, heartburn, appears more often in people who suffer excessive coughing from severe lung disease. Because this symptom is caused by the irritant

Symptoms associated with GERD	
Respiratory:	coughing
	wheezing
	bronchopneumonia
	apneic (non-breathing) episodes (in infants)
Gastrointestinal:	nausea
	vomiting
	dyspepsia (indigestion)
	abdominal pain/heartburn
	decreased appetite
Malnutrition	

effect of the acid, one very effective way of treating the condition is to use antacids to neutralize the acid. This works quite well if the heartburn comes and goes. If the problem is prolonged, though, or is present on a regular basis, there are at least two types of medicine that will very effectively inhibit the production of stomach acid.

The Pancreas

The pancreas has two distinct functions in the digestive process. The first is to produce and secrete enzymes to digest the proteins and fats in our food. Its second, very important function is to produce and secrete insulin, a hormone, into the bloodstream. Insulin controls the level of sugar that's been absorbed into the bloodstream as part of the digestive process, largely by controlling how much sugar is absorbed by various cells in the body. Without insulin, the body can't readily take up sugar and can't use the sugar for normal energy production.

Pancreatic Insufficiency

One of the most striking features of CF results from maldigestion (faulty digestion) and malabsorption (faulty absorption) of fats, which occur because the pancreas doesn't function normally (*pancreatic insufficiency*). Most of the enzymes necessary for the digestion of fats and proteins are produced within the pancreas, and are secreted into the ducts that drain the pancreas into the small intestine. In CF the secretions become thick and block the duct system (remember, the CFTR is absent from duct-lining cells, and the secretions produced within the ducts will be unusually thick). These abnormally thick secretions obstruct the normal flow of enzymes, which damages those cells of the pancreas concerned with enzyme production. The damaged pancreatic cells are then gradually replaced by scar tissue. As a result, not enough enzymes are produced, and any enzymes produced by the remaining cells can't reach the small intestine. Because the lipases don't reach the small intestine in adequate amounts, fats aren't digested properly and can't be absorbed. These undigested fats pass through the intestines and form the bulky, greasy and foul-smelling stools that are so characteristic of CF.

Similarly, proteases can't get to the small intestine to digest protein, which we need for normal growth and repair of body tissue. As a result of this maldigestion of protein and fat, growth slows down and malnutrition may develop.

Enzymes that will restore normal digestion are available in capsule form, but they must be taken with every meal and every snack. The type and amount of enzymes taken vary from person to person; it's a matter of trial and error, trying different combinations and quantities of the medications and seeing how they affect the stools. The goal is to produce one to two normal or near normal bowel movements per day. This very important aspect of CF treatment will be dealt with in more detail in Chapter 9.

Diabetes

The cells in the pancreas that produce the insulin hormone are called islet cells. The insulin produced by these cells is secreted directly into the bloodstream and doesn't have to pass through the duct system to be effective. The islet cells seem to be very tough; they survive and function even when the pancreas has been quite damaged by CF. It is only when destruction of the pancreas is very advanced that not enough insulin is produced. When that happens, cells in the body can't take up and metabolize sugar, so blood sugar levels rise. This, of course, is known as diabetes. About 15 percent of all people with CF will develop diabetes at some point, and they'll need to be treated with insulin to control their blood sugar levels. Diabetes is covered in more detail later in this chapter.

Pancreatitis

Occasionally, in those patients (up to 15 percent) who do have pancreatic enzyme production, localized inflammation occurs as the enzymes attack the pancreatic tissue. This produces intense pain in the upper abdomen, and sometimes nausea and vomiting. Pancreatic enzymes can actually leak out of the inflamed tissue and can be detected in the bloodstream, which

CF and the pancreas, esophagus, stomach and intestines

Organ	Condition	Percentage of CF patients affected
Pancreas	pancreatic insufficiency	85%
	diabetes	15%
	pancreatitis	15%
Esophagus, stomach	reflux, heartburn	10–20%
	ulcers	1–10%
Intestines	meconium ileus	10%
	rectal prolapse	10–20%
	fibrosing colonopathy	1%
	distal intestinal obstruction syndrome	10–20%
	intussusception	1%

aids in diagnosing this condition. Treatment may include stopping all feeding and providing intravenous nutrition for several days, until the inflammation subsides and the pain resolves.

Pancreatitis appears to be much more common in older age groups, and is very seldom seen in infancy and childhood.

The Stomach and Small Intestines

People with cystic fibrosis occasionally develop peptic ulcer symptoms, because they appear to secrete higher than normal amounts of acid from the stomach. This increased acidity would normally be neutralized by the digestive secretions from the pancreas, but, as we saw, pancreatic function is reduced in most people with CF, which allows the acid to remain very active in the small intestine, and particularly in its first section, the duodenum. The result is ulceration in the wall of the duodenum. When this happens, the person will usually complain of pain in the upper abdomen, just below the ribs and lower end of the breastbone. Ulcers are usually diagnosed by inserting a telescope-like instrument called a *gastroscope* into the stomach and duodenum, which allows us to see the ulceration. Treatment involves controlling the amount of acid produced by the stomach, which can be done with the same medications we use to treat acid reflux symptoms.

The Small and Large Intestines

Distal Intestinal Obstruction Syndrome (DIOS)

Meconium ileus, the most common form of obstruction in the newborn infant, was discussed in Chapter 1. Older people may develop a type of bowel obstruction called *distal intestinal obstruction syndrome*, or DIOS. This appears to be the adult equivalent of meconium ileus, and in the past was referred to as *meconium ileus equivalent*, or MIE. We still don't know how or why this occurs, though it may be because the intestinal mucus becomes very thick and, as the thickened secretions accumulate within the small bowel, they form an obstruction. Obstructions are especially likely to happen where the small intestine narrows at the entry point of the large intestine. Other factors can make the mucus thicker—becoming dehydrated, or not taking enough enzymes, or changing the diet to include foods that contain a lot of fiber—and contribute to the development of intestinal obstructions. DIOS symptoms begin as colicky or crampy abdominal pain; severe symptoms can also include distension of the abdomen, loss of appetite and even vomiting. Correcting this condition can be as simple as using an enema to empty the bowel of all of its contents. Another effective method is to ingest a solution of polyethylene glycol, which acts as an internal lubricant that helps the obstructing stool slide through the bowel more smoothly.

How CF affects the digestive system

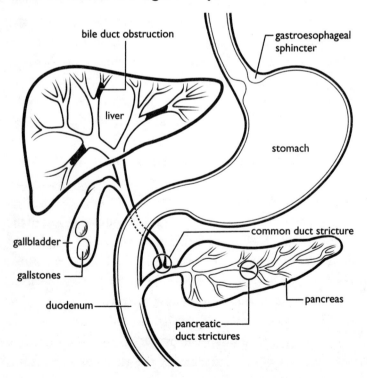

Intussusception

An intussusception is another form of bowel obstruction. It occurs when a portion of the bowel (usually the end of the small bowel) folds or slides into the large bowel, much the way an extended telescope slides into itself. When this happens, it interferes with blood flow in the telescoped part of the bowel, causing that part to swell. The result is an intestinal obstruction in that area. Bleeding may occur, and the blood may be passed from the rectum. The symptoms resemble those of DIOS. This condition can be easily diagnosed by an abdominal ultrasound examination, CT examination, or special abdominal X-rays using air or dye-containing enemas. Sometimes the air or enema itself pushes the telescoped bowel back to its normal position. If it doesn't, surgery may be required to relieve the obstruction.

Rectal Prolapse

This has also been discussed in Chapter 1. Although we see it mostly in children between one and three years old, it sometimes happens in adults as well. Straining when trying to pass stools because of constipation, bulky stools that tend toward diarrhea, and malnutrition can all predispose a person to developing this condition. Rectal prolapse will usually correct itself once the underlying problems are treated, but if it persists, the prolapse can be passed back gently into the rectum with a finger. Sometimes a persistent or recurrent prolapse needs to be stitched back into place by a small surgical procedure.

Fibrosing Colonopathy

In the early 1990s, some people with CF, primarily Europeans, developed multiple and very severe strictures, or narrowings, of their large bowels. These people tended to use enzyme supplements with very high lipase contents, so these enzyme preparations were taken off the market. We now know that very high doses of enzymes are possibly harmful. However, with careful use of the enzyme supplements currently available, fibrosing colonopathy doesn't appear to be a significant problem.

The Liver

The bile salts that the liver contributes to the digestive process are found in bile, a liquid produced by liver cells and secreted into the bile ducts. The bile then drains into the gallbladder and is stored until it's used during digestion. After we eat a meal, the gallbladder contracts and empties bile through the common bile duct into the small intestine, where the bile is mixed with the food passing from the stomach. The duct system in the liver is also lined by cells that lack the normal CFTR; as a result, the bile secretions become thickened and may block all those duct systems. Although liver cells may be damaged by the bile obstruction, the liver appears to be relatively more resistant to damage than the pancreas.

Changes to the liver appear in about 25 percent of the CF population, but people often aren't aware of these changes because they don't always produce noticeable symptoms. It's not clear what the long-term effects of liver changes may be, or what may develop as people with CF live longer and longer. At present, however, only about 2 to 10 percent will ever develop symptoms suggestive of liver disease; males tend to be affected more than females.

Prolonged Neonatal Jaundice

It's not unusual for newborn babies to develop some jaundice (yellowish color of the skin) in the first few days of life. This color comes from bilirubin, which is produced during the

CF and the liver

Condition	Percentage of CF patients affected
Bile duct stenosis	1–2%
Prolonged neonatal jaundice	5%
Fatty infiltration	20–60%
Focal biliary fibrosis	10–60%
Cirrhosis	1–25%
Portal hypertension	5–30%

body's normal daily recycling of red blood cells. This recycling occurs within the liver, and the bilirubin produced is excreted into the intestines in the bile. After birth, when the liver begins to function better, this yellow coloring in the skin fades away as the liver removes the bilirubin from the bloodstream. Occasionally, in CF newborns, the bile ducts become filled with a very thick sludge of bile and other materials. As a result, the removal of bilirubin is delayed, and the baby looks jaundiced for longer than most newborns. Fortunately the liver does eventually manage to pass this material through the ducts and function normally. Once this happens, the bilirubin is cleared from the baby's body and the jaundice gradually fades. This may take up to six months, but it generally clears completely, without any lasting effects.

Fatty Infiltration of the Liver

The most common change noticed in the liver is simply enlargement, and this can be detected by a physical examination of the abdomen. Very often, no symptoms are present even when the liver is quite enlarged. The enlargement occurs as the liver cells become filled with and distended by fat. While we don't know for sure what causes this, it does appear to be more common in people who become malnourished as a result of a poor diet. Although few newborns have enlarged livers, up to 10 percent of people with CF may have this condition by the time they're twenty.

Focal Biliary Fibrosis

This name refers to localized (focal) scarring (fibrosis) of the bile (biliary) system. When the flow of bile through the bile ducts draining the liver gets obstructed, the liver tissue surrounding those ducts becomes damaged, and scar tissue forms, increasing over time. Because this is a result of the defect of CFTR, just as we've seen in the lung and pancreas, it will probably occur to some degree in everyone with CF. The development of this scarring rarely produces symptoms, and no treatment is required unless blood tests indicate ongoing damage to the liver (see the section on ursodeoxycholic acid, below).

Cirrhosis

Continued obstruction of the bile flow from the liver may lead to further damage within the liver tissue itself. As the amount of fibrosis gradually increases, it distorts the structure of the liver, and this damage is called *cirrhosis*. Once cirrhosis has started, it tends to get worse and eventually it may interfere with the normal functioning of the liver. In fact, very severe cirrhosis can cause liver failure. The scarring process has another major detrimental effect: it prevents normal blood flow within the liver. As this occurs, blood is diverted and passes through other venous channels in the body called *varices*. These abnormal blood channels tend to bleed, and the bleeding most often happens in the stomach, which will show up as vomiting of blood. Scarring prevents normal blood flow out of the spleen as well. The spleen, an organ involved in the production of red blood cells, becomes enlarged, and this too can be felt when examining the abdomen. The scarring also prevents normal blood flow from the small intestines through the portal vein into the liver. The result is increased pressure in this vein, which is called portal hypertension.

How Do We Monitor Liver Function?

Liver Function Tests
When liver cells are damaged, they release enzymes into the bloodstream. These enzymes are easily detected by simple blood tests that can be used to monitor the severity of the problem. Tests should be done once a year, or more often if the liver is being actively affected.

Ultrasound Examination
Ultrasound can be used to show whether the liver is enlarged, and can also provide information on the kinds of changes happening in the liver—for example, whether there's fatty infiltration, or whether cirrhosis has developed. It can also be used to detect enlargement of the spleen.

Liver Biopsy
When there's any question about the diagnosis of liver enlargement or of a liver abnormality based on ultrasound examination or a CT scan, the doctor may order a biopsy. Biopsies involve introducing a special biopsy needle through the skin to extract a small sample of liver tissue, or may require a small incision. This test is not done very often.

What Can Be Done If Liver Changes Are Found?

Ursodeoxycholic Acid
Ursodeoxycholic acid (UDCA) is used to treat people who have elevated liver enzymes in the bloodstream. It's a form of bile acid that the liver can absorb and excrete into the bile in addition to the person's own bile acids, which are thought to be toxic to liver cells. When people are started on UDCA, their liver function does appear to normalize, so it appears that UDCA helps the liver cells. However, it's not clear yet whether this substance will continue to work over a long period of time.

Nutrition
It seems that malnutrition contributes significantly to the development of fatty infiltration of the liver. For this reason, people with this condition should have their eating habits reviewed at a clinic, and should promptly make any changes that the staff suggest.

Transplantation of the Liver
Occasionally, despite treatment, cirrhosis of the liver gets worse. When this happens and liver failure develops, or when symptoms of portal hypertension appear, a liver transplant may need to be considered.

The Gallbladder

Nonfunctioning Gallbladder and Micro Gallbladder
Some people with CF have smaller than normal gallbladders—a condition known as micro gallbladder. As well, some have nonfunctioning gallbladders; the gallbladder does not appear to store bile in a normal fashion, and does not con-

CF and the gallbladder

Condition	Percentage of CF patients affected
Nonfunctioning and micro gallbladder	12–40%
Gallstones	25%
Cholecystitis	5%

tract to empty bile into the small intestine during normal digestion. We don't know why these conditions occur. Most often, they just happen to be noted in the course of investigations for abdominal complaints or pain, or during the investigation of liver disease. Neither condition usually causes any symptoms.

Gallstones

Gallstones are small, hard masses that sometimes form in the gallbladder. People with CF get gallstones more often than people without the disorder. About one in ten in the CF population will develop them, and the incidence appears to increase with age. Typically the person experiences sharp, intermittent or colicky pain in the right upper part of the abdomen; removing the gallbladder will almost certainly cure the condition. This can usually be done quite easily, with minimal surgery, through a telescope-like instrument called a *laparoscope*.

Inflammation of the Gallbladder (Cholecystitis)

Occasionally there is colicky pain similar to gallstone pain, but doctors can't find any gallstones. In cases like this, inflammation of the gallbladder is thought to be the culprit. Like gallstones, this condition is more common in people with CF, and surgical removal of the gallbladder will cure it.

Diabetes

Daniel had enjoyed relatively good health since being diagnosed with CF when he was two. Through careful regulation
of his diet and the use of pancreatic enzymes with each
meal, he had managed to achieve normal height and weight.
Throughout his childhood he was able to participate in
all school activities without practically no difficulty. When
he transferred to the adult CF clinic at the age of eighteen he
had very few physical complaints, but he did admit to coughing on a daily basis and producing small amounts of yellowish sputum.

One day, about six months later, he complained of slowly
increasing fatigue over the previous two months. He said
that for a week or two he had been drinking about ten glasses
of fluids per day, and passing very large amounts of urine as
well. When clinic staff weighed him, they noted that he'd lost
sixteen pounds (over 7 kilos) since his previous visit. His
blood sugar was three times normal, and a spot test showed
sugar in his urine. Further testing confirmed CF-related diabetes mellitus, and Daniel was sent immediately to an
endocrinologist. He attended a diabetic education clinic
within days of his diagnosis, and was started on insulin injections to control his blood sugar. In addition, a dietitian
reviewed his diet and made minor changes to help control
his blood sugar.

Within several weeks, Daniel's blood sugar was stabilized
at normal levels and he had regained five pounds. He soon felt
his usual self, and he was able to accept a full-time job that
he'd been considering, but he continues to take insulin twice
a day.

Diabetes is now seen in about 15 percent of all people with
CF. Although children don't usually develop it, the incidence

of diabetes increases as they get older. Diabetes appears to affect only those who have true pancreatic insufficiency and need enzyme replacement for normal digestion. Diabetes can be brought on by drugs that interfere with glucose (sugar) metabolism, such as corticosteroids, or as a result of increasing nutrition by such methods as intravenous (IV) feeding (see Chapter 9).

Is Diabetes the Same in People with CF?

You may have heard about diabetics who develop the disease at an early age and need insulin to keep their blood sugar under good control. You may also have heard about a different form of diabetes that appears in later life and doesn't require insulin; this late-onset type can be managed with a combination of diet and drugs that either stimulate insulin secretion by the pancreas, or help cells in the body make better use of the insulin available. The person with CF who also has diabetes seems to fall somewhere between these two types. In the CF person, the onset of diabetes appears to be milder and much slower. It tends to produce fewer symptoms and also tends to be associated with fewer of the usual complications. As well, the later complications so common with diabetics don't appear to develop as early or as severely. However, as the CF population lives longer, those with diabetes may develop more physical complications. Only time will tell how varied or how severe these complications will be.

When Do We Suspect Diabetes?

Often, people with CF come in to the clinic with very ill-defined complaints or symptoms. They may simply fail to gain weight as expected, or they may feel unduly tired or easily fatigued whenever they try to exercise. This is very likely due to the

Symptoms suggestive of diabetes

- excessive thirst, drinking fluids
- excessive urination
- unexplained weight loss
- blurred vision

inability of the cells of the body to take up sugar from the blood normally for energy production.

If the blood sugar rises high enough, it's removed from the body by the kidneys, which excrete the excess sugar into the urine. This results in very large volumes of urine being produced daily. As this water is excreted, the person becomes dehydrated and feels extremely thirsty. He or she ends up drinking huge quantities of water—another characteristic symptom of the untreated diabetic. As dehydration increases, changes occur in the eye and the person will complain of blurred vision—another characteristic symptom of diabetes.

How Do We Diagnose Diabetes?

Blood Sugar
Diabetes is indicated by the presence of high levels of blood sugar when the patient has fasted overnight and has blood drawn and tested early in the morning. When this *fasting level* is greater than 7.8 millimoles per liter of blood, or 126 milligrams per deciliter—7.8 mmol/L or 126 mg/dL—a diagnosis of diabetes is very likely. If the patient has the symptoms of diabetes described above, the diagnosis can be accepted. If the person has no symptoms, the fasting blood sugar test will likely be repeated to confirm the diagnosis.

Urine Testing
Diabetes may also be suspected when sugar is detected in the urine. This usually happens only when the blood sugar levels are very high.

Treatment of Diabetes

Diet
Keeping to a proper diet is a mainstay of diabetes treatment. Someone with CF who has been diagnosed as diabetic *must* go over his or her diet with a qualified dietitian, to ensure a proper, balanced meal plan to help maintain overall well-being. While there will probably not be any major changes to the usual high-energy CF diet, it will likely be best to avoid readily absorbed simple sugars such as candy products or soft drinks, which can make controlling blood sugars more difficult than it need be.

Pills That Lower Blood Sugar
These *oral hypoglycemic agents* work by stimulating the small insulin-producing cells in the pancreas to secrete more insulin. They tend to be used to treat the mild diabetic, and they are very often all that is necessary for a diabetic person with CF.

Insulin
The most efficient way to treat diabetes is through injections of insulin. This supplies the body with the insulin it needs daily for normal sugar metabolism, and replaces the insulin that the destroyed islet cells can no longer produce. Once it's been decided that someone needs insulin to control blood sugar, it's unlikely that he or she will ever be able to stop taking it.

Insulin is a fairly effective treatment for diabetes, but it requires careful adjustment of doses to diet, and constant monitoring. The many aspects of using insulin are beyond the scope of this book. Anyone using insulin should be working with a diabetic health-care team. As well, there are helpful books available that treat this complex subject comprehensively.

CF and the Reproductive System

s people with CF approach adulthood, they face a series of major changes in their lives. Most strikingly, their concerns shift away from the family home to very personal issues, such as choosing a career, furthering education (perhaps to the university level and beyond), forming lasting relationships and maybe even marriage. As they develop their own unique identities and relationships, some will eventually consider parenthood. While parenthood is a major decision for both men and women with CF, it has more impact on the women. To understand the issues that may arise, we need to review the effects of CF on the male and female reproductive systems.

Are CF Males Different from CF Females?

The obvious answer is yes, they are. However, CF females have reproductive organs that appear normal in structure, while changes occur in males that are specific to CF itself.

The testicles in males with CF develop in the usual way, so that they appear normal in both structure and function. The testicles have two purposes: to produce sperm, and to create the hormone testosterone, which they discharge into the bloodstream. Testosterone generates secondary male sexual characteristics such as increased body hair, growth and maturation of the testicles, deepening of the voice and, above all, sexual drive and interest. Because the testicles function normally in CF males, all of these functions develop normally also, so that men can function in a sexual relationship like anyone else.

However, having CF does result in one very important change for a man. It involves the epididymides, which normally collect the sperm produced in the testicles, and the collecting tubules and vas deferens, through which the sperm are pumped out, or ejaculated, during sexual activity. These structures may be absent even as early as birth—the only obvious physical abnormality in the newborn male. Although we don't know why this occurs, it probably happens for the same reason that liver and pancreas ducts become blocked up. Once the collecting ducts or tubules are destroyed, the sperm can no longer get out of the body. This damage affects 95 percent of CF males, which is why so few of them are able to father children. Remember, however, that approximately 5 percent

Congenital bilateral absence of the vas deferens (CBAVD)

This is a similar condition that appears in men who do not show other characteristics of cystic fibrosis. We're aware of it because it's now fairly easy to do genetic testing. A small group of men who went to fertility clinics because they couldn't father children turned out to have CBAVD. The men did not appear to have any physical problems until researchers noticed that they lacked the collecting system so often missing in men with CF. When the researchers examined the men's genes, they found that the men had gene defects seen in cystic fibrosis. This small group of men seemed to have either a very mild form of cystic fibrosis, or perhaps a different type of CF that we still don't know much about.

of men with CF do produce sperm normally and can ejaculate it successfully. As a result, this small proportion are able to father children.

Can Anything Correct This Abnormality?

At present there's no simple way to correct the defect. Unfortunately, the ducts are destroyed and can't be replaced. Very specialized centers have attempted to remove sperm directly from the testicle with a needle, and use them to artificially fertilize eggs taken from the female partner through in-vitro fertilization; if a sperm fertilizes an egg, the fertilized egg is then placed inside the woman's uterus at the time she could normally conceive. If the procedure is successful, the egg implants as in a normal pregnancy and develops into a normal fetus. Unfortunately for the would-be parents, these techniques have a very low success rate and are very expensive. Very often the couple themselves have to pay these high costs. However, a man with CF who wants to father a child has little other choice.

It's important to counsel and educate boys about all this as they are going through puberty, so that they understand their physical problem and realize that, as a result, they may never be able to father children.

The Female Reproductive System

The female reproductive organs include the uterus, the fallopian tubes and the ovaries. In a woman with CF there are no specific abnormalities in any of these organs, unlike the changes in the male reproductive system. The ovaries, like the testicles in the male, have two main functions. They produce the ovum, or egg, once a month as a part of the normal menstrual cycle, and release it into the fallopian tube for possible fertilization. As well, the ovaries release the hormones estrogen and progesterone, which generate secondary female sexual characteristics like growth of body hair and breast development. These hormones also prepare the uterus for pregnancy each month, which results in the normal monthly cycle of menstruation.

Reproductive Problems in Women with CF

Delayed Menstruation
Menarche, or the onset of menstruation, occurs about two years later than average in females with CF. Menarche usually happens at about twelve and a half years of age in North America, but may not occur in girls with CF until fourteen and a half. We don't know the reason for this delay. An ongoing illness such as severe lung disease may be the cause. Nutrition may also play a role.

Difficulties with Menstruation
Problems with menstruation are more common even in women who are only mildly affected by CF. Up to 50 percent of women with CF have menstrual periods that are irregular in duration, and menstrual flows that are scanty and irregular. Menstrual irregularities may increase if they develop significant malnutrition or if their lung disease gets worse. If the degree of malnutrition or lung disease worsens even further, menstrual flow may disappear completely—a condition called *amenorrhea*.

Issues with Pregnancy
Despite the fact that women with CF have normal reproductive systems, becoming pregnant may pose a real and significant problem. As a group, such women appear to be relatively infertile—that is, they have difficulty becoming pregnant, probably because of thick mucus in the cervix. Just as defects in the

CFTR protein cause abnormal mucus production in the airways of the lungs, defective CFTR protein in the cells lining the cervical canal may cause similarly abnormally thick mucus which plugs the entrance to the uterus and prevents sperm from entering, forming a type of internal contraception. This does not affect all women with CF to the same degree; many have been able to become pregnant and to experience normal pregnancies and births. Occasionally, if this mucous barrier is preventing pregnancy, a physician (usually an obstetrician/gynecologist) can help by inserting a sperm specimen from the partner directly into the uterus at the appropriate time in the menstrual cycle (i.e., by artificial insemination).

Twenty-three years old and newly married to Jason, Gloria arrived for a routine CF clinic follow-up and asked to discuss the possibility of starting a family, and how a pregnancy might affect her. She was in good health, and had kept her body weight within normal limits through enzyme supplements and careful attention to her diet. Her lung function was within 75 percent of expected values for her age. Because her lung function didn't appear to be a problem, the doctor referred Gloria and Jason to a medical geneticist—a specialist in the diagnosis of and counseling for genetic diseases—for further review. Jason underwent genetic testing for the common CF gene defects, and happily none was detected. After careful genetic counseling to point out that all Gloria's children would be carriers of the CF gene, Gloria and her husband were told it was very unlikely that they'd have a child with cystic fibrosis. Several months later, Gloria announced that she was pregnant. Her CF doctor and the CF clinic dietitian monitored her closely and made sure she maintained her weight throughout her pregnancy. Gloria had a normal labor and delivered a healthy baby girl.

Should Women with CF Get Pregnant?

All CF women considering pregnancy should seek counseling and advice before proceeding, and this should be done very early in a relationship. The counseling is important for several reasons. The woman and her partner should clearly understand the risks of pregnancy to the woman, and the possible consequences to the child, who may carry the CF gene or even have the disease itself. Fortunately, in this day and age, the partner's genes can be checked before he undertakes such a responsibility. Remember from Chapter 3 that, if the partner of a woman with CF carries the CF gene, all the children will be affected in some way; each child will have a fifty-fifty chance of having CF versus being a carrier of the abnormal CF gene.

Both partners should also realize that the CF mother faces an average life expectancy of between thirty-six and thirty-seven years. She must be prepared for the very real possibility that she may never see her children reach adulthood, and may never be able to participate in the many things that parents normally look forward to as their children grow up.

Pregnancy may have a significant effect on both the mother-to-be and the developing baby. Both partners should recognize that:

- pregnancy may be detrimental to the health of the mother
- the developing fetus may be adversely affected by the state of the mother's health
- breast-feeding may adversely affect the health of the mother

What Is the Effect of Pregnancy on the Mother?

Many changes in body function occur as pregnancy progresses. The burden of providing for another, rapidly growing life within the womb puts added stress on the heart, lungs and nutritional status of the mother. Pregnancy by itself does not appear to produce any significant or harmful effects upon the mother's lung function, nor does it appear to have any adverse

Signs that a woman with CF should avoid pregnancy

- FEV_1 below 50 percent of expected value
- blood oxygen less than 60 mmHg
- blood carbon dioxide greater than 45 mmHg
- swelling of ankles (indicating strain of the right side of the heart)
- body weight below 70 percent of expected weight
- significant liver disease
- possibly, CF-related diabetes (still controversial)

effect upon her life expectancy, provided that she is well prior to the pregnancy.

Pregnancy is generally safe if the mother's CF remains relatively mild. If she scores better than 60 percent of predicted values on pulmonary function tests such as the FEV_1, the pregnancy will usually go very well. Likewise, if her chest X-ray shows only very mild changes and if she is above 70 percent of her ideal body weight, the pregnancy will likely go well.

However, the mother needs to consume as much as 10 percent more calories to maintain the pregnancy, and this may be a problem for a woman with CF. Someone with CF usually requires 20 to 30 percent more calories than other people simply to maintain good nutrition; it may be a major feat for a CF mother to maintain adequate nutrition throughout a pregnancy. Mothers who are malnourished, or who become so during the pregnancy, are much more likely to deliver their babies too soon, and to have babies with low birth weights. Even if the newborn is genetically normal, these two factors can cause severe breathing problems for the baby at birth, and a greater risk of death in infancy.

What Are the Effects of CF on the Baby?
The baby will experience no adverse effects from the mother's CF as long as the mother stays in good overall health. Most pregnancies last the full nine months, and a normal delivery

usually occurs, without any unusual complications. Doctors must be cautious about prescribing medication to the CF mother during this period, but the medications commonly used in the day-to-day management of CF do not pose any significant risk for the baby. Acute respiratory infections during pregnancy may need antibiotic treatment, but most antibiotics used are safe for both mother and baby. Antibiotics like streptomycin, trimethoprim, sulfonamides of all types, tetracyclines of all types and chloramphenicol should be avoided. Fortunately, doctors seldom prescribe these antibiotics for patients with CF, and safe alternatives are available. At present, fluoroquinolones are avoided in pregnancy, because of potential damage to developing cartilage in the baby. Although the only evidence for this comes from animal studies, until we can be sure that fluoroquinolones are safe for use in pregnant women, they shouldn't take them at all. Again, other safe antibiotics are available to substitute for the fluoroquinolones.

Breast-feeding

CF mothers may very well want to breast-feed their newborn infants. They can be reassured that CF doesn't have any effect upon either the content or the quantity of maternal milk. The major concern is the added energy demands that breast-feeding places on the mother, in terms of overall nutrition. She will need an additional 500 calories per day to produce the milk normally needed for breast-feeding. She must be very careful to allow for this, and must be able to consume all these extra calories. Most CF drugs can cross to the newborn through the mother's milk, but this is not an issue, as they pose no significant risks. However, the antibiotics noted above as a concern during pregnancy can also be passed through the mother's milk. When breast-feeding, mothers should avoid all of those antibiotics.

Complications associated with pregnancy

Complication	Percent affected
miscarriage	21%
pre-term delivery	27%

Birth Control

Males

Since 5 percent of men with CF are capable of fathering children, all CF males should have their semen analyzed, probably at about the time they shift from pediatric to adult care. As young men become sexually active they should always be aware of the consequences of their actions, and of what chance they have of fathering children. Those males with CF who are capable of fathering children should use contraceptives to prevent unwanted pregnancies.

Females

Despite the fact that women with CF tend to be relatively infertile, they should not assume that they will have difficulty conceiving. If they are sexually active, they should use some form of contraception. Acceptable methods include:

- hormonal contraceptives
- barrier methods such as a diaphragm with a spermicidal agent
- condom use by the partner, along with a spermicidal agent
- tubal ligation ("tying the tubes")

Intra-uterine devices (IUDs) have caused unwanted side effects in women with CF. They should be avoided.

S I X

Unusual Manifestations of CF

B y far the major manifestations of cystic fibrosis involve the lungs, the digestive system and the reproductive system, covered in the preceding chapters. There are also some rather uncommon problems, however, which we'll look at in this chapter.

Problems of Bones and Joints

Osteoporosis

When Kelly was transferred to the adult cystic fibrosis clinic at age eighteen, she had already been admitted several times to the children's hospital for recurring chest infections. She told the adult-clinic staff that, in addition to her symptoms of daily cough and sputum production, she'd been getting pain in her ankles and hips. The pain occurred every two or three months and usually went away with pain medication. Her doctor reassured her that this was not uncommon in people with CF. He added that it might be due, in part, to a weakening of her bones as a result of the disorder—also fairly common in people with CF as they grew older. He explained that the clinic routinely got a DEXA scan on all new patients. (DEXA is short for dual energy X-ray absorptiometry.) This scan measured the density of bone, which gave an idea of the strength of that bone as well. He said that the test was very much like a simple X-ray exam. It would take only fifteen to twenty minutes, and all Kelly had to do was lie on a scanning table while the camera in the scanner measured the density of bone in her hip joint and in the vertebrae of her lower spine.

The scan showed that Kelly's bones weren't as dense or as strong as they should be at her age. To strengthen her bones and to prevent further loss of bone strength, and in the hope of preventing fractures, Kelly's doctor put her on vitamin D supplements and calcium tablets. Arrangements were made to repeat the bone scan in twelve to eighteen months, to make sure that the therapy was working and that no further deterioration was occurring.

Osteoporosis is a bone disease characterized by a reduced bone mass (bone density), which results from deterioration of the fine structure of the bone tissue. Bone is a living tissue that's constantly being resorbed, remodeled and rebuilt by small cells within it. New bone growth continues until we've achieved our full growth potential in our late teens. Bone is then remodeled and repaired throughout our lives. Calcium plays an important part in this process, because calcium is incorporated into all new bone growth, and is used in remodeling bone, to give it strength.

Between thirty and forty years of age, we begin to lose bone mass, and we lose about 3 to 5 percent every ten years. As bone loss occurs, the bone looks porous or full of holes—hence the name osteoporosis (osteo = bone, porous = full of holes). This makes the bone more fragile and subject to fractures. Osteoporosis becomes much more common with advancing age.

Factors contributing to the development of osteoporosis

- poor absorption of vitamin D and calcium from the digestive tract
- malnutrition
- genetic factors
- hypogonadism (low testosterone in males and low estrogen in females)
- reduced physical activity
- prolonged use of corticosteroids such as prednisone
- use of cyclosporin (by transplant patients)
- diabetes
- chronic infection
- severe CF disease

Osteoporosis has also come to be recognized as a significant problem for the adolescent and adult with CF—in fact, it appears to be present in virtually all who survive to early adulthood. As the person approaches adulthood, bone development may be deficient and the bones don't seem to be as strong as they would be in a normal individual. Even a healthy-looking person with CF is likely to have osteoporosis. The cause of CF-related osteoporosis may be related to a variety of factors.

In people with CF, the most significant contributing factor in the development of osteoporosis appears to be malnutrition. Although malnutrition may be an issue at any age, it becomes a particular problem in older people, for whom respiratory problems are more common and more intense. As lung disease progresses, appetite usually decreases, food intake declines and malnutrition may result.

Another major reason for osteoporosis may be poor absorption of vitamin D and calcium. Vitamin D must be dissolved in digested fat before it can be absorbed from the gastrointestinal tract. If the fats are not absorbed, any dissolved vitamin D will not be absorbed either.

Oral corticosteroid preparations can also contribute to osteoporosis. People who have undergone transplants are especially susceptible, because they have to take corticosteroids daily to prevent rejection of the transplanted organ.

Diagnosis of Osteoporosis
The degree of osteoporosis may be assessed by the DEXA scan, which measures the density of bones. If the bone mass is reduced, treatment should be undertaken to attempt to reverse this process.

Treatment of Osteoporosis
Treatment includes the following steps:
- Nutritional deficiencies should be addressed and corrected as much as possible.
- Supplemental vitamin D and calcium should be taken, in pill form. (Some doctors consider that treatment with vitamin D and calcium should start at puberty, even if the DEXA scan is normal.)
- If the DEXA scan shows the osteoporosis to be severe, drugs that prevent calcium from being removed from bone (which occurs in everyone on a day-to-day basis, as part of the body's normal metabolism) may be prescribed. These drugs are called *bisphosphonates* and are most easily taken orally.

Why Treat Osteoporosis?
Treatment of osteoporosis is especially important for people with CF because they have a higher incidence of spontaneous fractures than do unaffected individuals. For example, spontaneous rib fractures occur very commonly and appear to be associated with severe bouts of coughing. Fractures of the ankle or the wrist seem to happen with very little in the way

of stress to the limb. Very often, in fact, osteoporosis is first suspected when one of these fractures occurs.

Prevention of Osteoporosis

Preventing osteoporosis is always more successful than trying to correct it once it's developed. Just as there are several ways in which osteoporosis can develop, there are several ways to try to prevent it. These include:

- maintaining adequate nutrition and good body weight
- ensuring that the diet contains the recommended daily calcium requirement for the appropriate age group
- engaging in as much physical activity as possible
- monitoring vitamin D blood levels and remedying deficiencies with vitamin D supplements as needed
- using corticosteroid preparations with caution and at the lowest dose possible.

Sore Joints and Limbs

Periodic Arthritis or Arthralgia

Lucy entered high school with few complaints related to her cystic fibrosis. Because she had normal lung function, she was able to take part in several school activities, including the track and field team. One day, without any warning, she felt pain in her right knee and ankle. The pain became so intense when she moved her right leg that she had to stop track and field, and she decided to see her CF doctor. He couldn't find any obvious abnormalities in her knee or ankle, but he reassured Lucy that this pain was related to her cystic fibrosis, and that no damage to her joints was likely. Lucy started taking an anti-inflammatory medication to reduce any inflammation in the joints, and to relieve the pain.

The treatment did control Lucy's pain, and it gradually went away over the next ten days. She was able to stop the medication and return to all her school activities. The doctor told her that the joint symptoms might return from time to time, and that she could control them with the use of medication such as ibuprofen, without always having to notify the clinic. He added that she should contact the clinic if the joint symptoms persisted or changed in any way despite her taking medication as instructed.

Although joint symptoms are unusual in childhood CF, up to 8 percent of adults develop joint complaints, and they are most common between twenty and thirty years of age.

Knees, ankles, elbows, wrists, fingers, shoulders and hips are the joints most people complain about. The symptoms may occur only once, or they may recur, at irregular intervals. In most cases, no lasting damage appears to be done within the joint, so this doesn't appear to be a true type of arthritis. An episode like this is often referred to as arthralgia, which simply means discomfort around a joint. Most often, the condition can be treated with simple anti-inflammatory agents such as ASA, acetaminophen, ibuprofen or, occasionally, corticosteroids, if the pain becomes very severe or incapacitating.

Hypertrophic Pulmonary Osteoarthropathy (HPOA)

A similar condition, called hypertrophic pulmonary osteoarthropathy, may also cause pain or discomfort around the ends of the long bones, such as the forearms or the lower legs. Very often, simply squeezing the bone with medium pressure will hurt. HPOA appears to occur as the *periosteum*—the layer of tissue that forms the surface layer of bone—becomes thickened, perhaps because of some form of inflammation of the bone. We see HPOA most often in people who have relatively advanced lung disease, particularly those with low levels of oxygen in their bloodstream. Treatment for HPOA is similar to the treatment given for periodic joint pain, and anti-inflammatory agents provide the best pain relief.

Skin Rashes

Adult Skin Rashes

Like HPOA, skin rashes appear mostly in people with relatively severe lung disease. Rashes sometimes crop up at the same time as joint pain first appears. The rash, which is usually on the lower legs and nearly always below the knees, appears as painless, rounded spots, slightly raised above the skin surface, and dark red to purple in color. The spots are about the size of a pinhead, although, if the rash is severe, the spots may seem to blend into one another, producing larger spots up to the size of a pea. Although the rash may look frightening, it usually causes no particular harm and goes away on its own. There is no specific treatment for this condition.

Infant Skin Rashes

Infants may develop a dry, scaly rash that involves the diaper area, the skin around the mouth, and the upper arms and shoulders. It seems to be related to failure to thrive, or malnutrition, and is mostly due to nutritional deficiencies in fatty acids, proteins and perhaps zinc. Once nutritional problems have been corrected, this rash usually clears up quickly.

Pneumatosis Intestinalis

This rare bowel disorder is produced by very small pockets of air that appear to develop, for reasons we don't know, in the surface lining of the large bowel. It's mostly found by chance, and sometimes when an X-ray of the abdomen is done after a person complains of vague pain or discomfort. In most cases this condition simply goes away on its own. Occasionally it leads to the development of bowel obstructions, and in that case surgery is usually required to remove the area of the bowel that's become obstructed.

Kidney Stones

The kidneys in themselves don't appear to be affected by cystic fibrosis. However, adults with CF do seem to have more kidney stones than average. The stones appear to be produced by high levels of a mineral called oxalate in the blood, which results from the malabsorption that happens in people with pancreatic problems. Kidney stones can cause severe pain, felt at the side of the abdomen or flank, but most stones are passed spontaneously in the urine. If a stone lodges in a ureter—the duct that carries urine from the kidney to the bladder—it can be removed by literally smashing it with ultrasound—a procedure called a lithotripsy. Although this may sound horrible, most people feel very little discomfort, as the stone simply crumbles. If this procedure isn't available, a urologist may try to take the stone out by passing a probe with a wire snare into the ureter or bladder, and snaring the stone.

SEVEN

Problems of Adolescence and Adulthood

By the year 2000, 40 percent of people with CF were living past the age of eighteen. For most of them this brings a new purpose to life, with fresh directions to take and unaccustomed responsibilities to assume. As the child with cystic fibrosis enters adolescence, care and other daily activities begin to shift from a small, close-knit core of family members and CF care providers to include a larger and more complex set of people outside the family, leading the child to new interests, friends and activities. It's during this transition that conflicts arise between caregivers and adolescents with CF, as the young people take on their new roles. Teenagers generally go through a fairly stormy period (as all parents know), but for the chronically ill teen this period may be much more difficult, because of the limitations or restrictions a chronic illness imposes.

It seemed as if eighteen-year-old Curtis was making the transition to the adult CF clinic quite normally. He appeared for his first visit after making his own appointment and driving himself

---

Adolescence
- begins with puberty, ends in late teens or early twenties
- is a time when teens think they are invincible
- is a time of critical transition
- is a time to begin gaining a unique identity or "self"
- is a time to gain both emotional and physical independence from parents
- is a time to fit in with peers while coping with being different

---

to the clinic. However, from that very first contact with clinic staff, it was obvious that Curtis was unhappy. He had entered university at the insistence of his parents, despite his wish to take a shorter community college course in electronics, with the hope of eventually working as a repairman of electronic equipment. This resulted in continuing arguments with his parents, and a constant struggle to achieve even passing grades at school. While he was discussing the reasons for his unhappiness on subsequent clinic visits, it became apparent that Curtis was very angry and upset with his parents, and with clinic staff. He had read on a CF website that most CF males were sterile and not likely to be able to father children, and he felt angry that no one had discussed this with him in the past.

When Curtis was seen on a follow-up visit, he admitted to being depressed about this knowledge, and he remained angry that he had not been told sooner. Continuing conflicts with his parents over schooling only added to his frustration and anxiety, and his grades in school fell even further.

Kyra failed to keep her first three appointments at the adult CF clinic. The clinic staff noted that during her teenage years she had also missed several appointments at the pediatric CF clinic. When she finally did attend the adult clinic, it was only to obtain a repeat of her bronchodilator medication—which she admitted to using only irregularly, and only when she was feeling very short of breath. She and her divorced mother, who worked full time in order to support them, lived in a small rural community about forty-five minutes from the nearest CF clinic. Kyra dropped out of high school without finishing grade 10, after many warnings about smoking on the school grounds and about skipping classes. She had few close friends, because she was embarrassed to use her medications or take enzymes when she was with anyone. As a result, she felt lonely and isolated from her peers, and this only got worse when she dropped out of school. She admitted to neglecting her physiotherapy because she "had no time for it," and because her mother "always nagged her to do it."

When Kyra was seen at the clinic, she was obviously under-nourished and she weighed less than 75 percent of her expected weight. She refused to have blood drawn for tests, and wouldn't stay to have pulmonary function studies done. She did do an FEV_1 measurement in the outpatient clinic, and this revealed that her FEV_1 was only 50 percent of that expected for her age, indicating that her cystic fibrosis had had a moderately severe effect on her lungs.

As children enter adolescence, new issues arise that may significantly affect their care. An important aspect of this period, for all adolescents, is the need to develop independence and to form their own identities. Most teens with CF recognize the nature and severity of their illness, although they may try to deny their ill health. Not infrequently at this time, however, they refuse to allow parents to give them treatments and medications. Caregivers may need to cut them some slack for a while. It's natural for adolescents to be concerned about their personal appearance, and particularly about peer acceptance.

Although significant problems may arise during this period, making interaction difficult between teens and their parents and caregivers, remember that help is always available from both the pediatric and the adult-care staff. Luckily, as most adolescents mature, they do become more responsible for their own care. Eventually they enter adulthood with reasonable expectations about their role in society, and about how that role will be affected by their illness.

Transition to the Adult Clinic

Once it's certain that a child has CF, the child and family will have most of their patient contacts with a specialized CF care team, usually one providing pediatric care. When the family's living situation doesn't allow for such a team to deliver regular care and follow-up, the task may fall to the family doctor. The CF clinic will still organize regular follow-up appointments and support the family doctor in providing care.

During these early years, the children usually develop close relationships with all their CF team members. The prospect of ending these relationships when they're going through the often turbulent teenage years may cause a great deal of anxiety, not only for the teens but also for their parents and other family members! Despite this anxiety, and the occasional reluctance on the part of the adolescent or family to transfer care to an adult setting, it's appropriate to switch to an adult clinic by the age of eighteen. This involves a transition from a family-oriented caregiving situation to one in which the doctor and other team members deal directly, one on one, with the young person, who accepts more and more responsibility for his or her own care.

Since Curtis was having so much trouble dealing with his anger and depression, the clinic arranged regular visits for him to work out a plan to overcome these feelings. A visit with the psychiatric liaison nurse was arranged, to assess his degree of depression and to provide guidance on dealing with his parents' expectations. Curtis was reassured that there was nothing abnormal about his feelings, under the circumstances. Curtis then met with the CF social worker, who arranged to meet with his parents and try to resolve their problem over Curtis's choice of an occupation. Eventually this was resolved, and Curtis switched to a community college, where he did well. Both the CF physician and the nurse coordinator discussed Curtis's sexuality with him, over several clinic visits. He was told that, although he might not be able to father children, his sexual function would be entirely normal. Gradually his anger over this disappeared, and his anxieties about having a girlfriend or other significant relationship went away. He was reassured that he could discuss these problems with clinic staff at any time, and he was encouraged to phone the staff with any problems that he felt he needed help for.

As for Kyra, during her first contact with the adult CF clinic, staff reviewed her past activities briefly with her. She was told that if she attended the adult CF clinic, she would no longer be treated like a child. She would be treated as an adult, and she would have to behave like one. She would have to make her own follow-up appointments for each visit, and she was encouraged to attend the clinic regularly.

After several irregular follow-ups, Kyra appeared to be more receptive to the clinic staff and more responsive to being treated as an adult. An appointment was arranged with the CF social worker, who spent several visits counseling Kyra about prospects for work, and about perhaps returning to school. It was thought best for Kyra to live independently, so the social worker made arrangements for her to find her own place to live, and helped her find a job. With much encouragement from the clinic coor-

The goals of transition

- transfer care to adult-based medicine
- provide age-specific care for issues unique to or more common in the adult setting: dating, marriage, employment, education, financial considerations
- facilitate/coordinate referral to a lung transplant program
- introduce issues of terminal care

dinator, Kyra eventually accepted the seriousness of her condition and agreed not to smoke any more. Her friends were allowed to come along on clinic visits, for support. As they came to understand her problem, Kyra accepted her treatment plans and agreed to follow them more closely. She was encouraged to call the CF coordinator to discuss problems as they occurred. She was also reassured that, if she made the effort to call the staff, they would always make an effort to help her overcome any problem that arose.

What Are the Goals of the Adult CF Team?

These are the same as the goals of the pediatric CF team, but with a slight but very significant change in emphasis, toward achieving the following goals.

Developing a Trusting Relationship

A prime goal for this transition period is to maintain the trust that patient and family have developed with the pediatric care team. Transferring the patient from the pediatric to the adult setting means ending familiar relationships while beginning unfamiliar ones. It's important that the adult-clinic team members adopt a non-judgmental approach, to allow maturing patients to learn to make their own decisions regarding their health concerns and the many new problems that will come along.

Maintaining Optimal Health

Maintaining the young person's optimal health is the prime goal of the adult-care team members, even if it means that the young person must abandon or change life goals, whether they involve education, career or family, because of CF-related illness.

Achieving Maximum Independence

It is always the purpose of the adult-team members to have their patients assume responsibility for their own care. This means getting them to understand their disease and how it may affect their future, and to make informed decisions on their own, concerning not only treatment but other life choices as well.

Team members work to help their patients achieve their life goals. In addition they encourage them to continue to set higher goals for themselves, as long as these goals are realistic.

When Does This Transition Begin?

The pediatric care team initiates the transition process in the one to two years prior to the patient's eighteenth birthday. They will likely start by introducing the teen and the rest of the family to the adult-team coordinator. The coordinator will in turn introduce the teen to various team members, usually well in advance of the actual transfer to the adult clinic. As well, there may be orientation visits to the outpatient department, physiotherapy department and hospital wards where the patient may come to be admitted. This

---

Elements of transition

* a shift from family/child-oriented pediatric care to adult/individual-oriented care
* a shift from school environment to workplace
* a shift from home to community/social situations
* a shift from the nuclear family to friends and special partnerships

allows the person to become familiar with the physical settings for adult care, and to feel less anxious about the transfer process itself.

During this period, the pediatric care team will try to have the young person gradually assume a larger role in decision-making, hoping that the teen will be able to make most care decisions independently of other family members by the time of the transfer to the adult clinic.

Once the young person has transferred to the adult clinic, the staff will

- introduce the person to all CF team members
- review the past medical history with the person
- assess the severity of the disease and review the current medical care arrangements
- introduce potential treatment options not already in use, if appropriate—for example, transplantation
- evaluate the person's potential for independence as well as the current level of independent functioning
- review and modify doctor and patient appreciation of their respective roles, responsibilities and expectations regarding the disease
- establish ground rules and expectations for all aspects of care; these ground rules will be put in place with mechanisms to ensure that the person participates in his or her care by
  a) making all day-to-day phone calls for all aspects of continuing care to the clinic coordinator
  b) making all clinic appointments or cancellations personally when necessary
  c) understanding how to contact the CF doctor or clinic coordinator for more urgent or emergency medical situations
  d) understanding that adults with CF are responsible for their own care

e) understanding that parents accompanying a young person to the adult clinic for the first time will be expected to remain in the waiting room on subsequent visits when the young person needs to see a doctor or team member

f) coming to an agreement with the doctor about how much information (if any) to share with parents or significant others

g) understanding that once the transition has occurred, the person may not return to the pediatric clinic.

Very often, during the early transition period, young people and/or their families try to contact the pediatric care team during times of stress, such as episodes of increased symptoms or illness, or during stays in the hospital.

Working toward a Better Understanding of CF
According to the majority of adult CF clinics, as many as 50 percent of young people transferring to the clinic do not appreciate the number, nature or range of disabilities that may affect them, now that people are living longer with cystic fibrosis. During the early transition period, staff generally make an effort to review the more common disabilities, as well as the usual respiratory problems, including such things as CF-related diabetes, fertility problems, liver problems, unusual infections such as cepacia and many other issues.

Clinic staff have also found that as many as half of these patients aren't able to explain what medications they are on and why they are taking them. For this reason, they may review the medications, how to take them, and the reasons why they were prescribed.

New treatment options may be introduced at this time, depending on how far the disease has progressed. Issues that may be raised include such things as transplantation, the use

When to discuss end-of-life issues

- when the disease has progressed to the point where it is obvious that longer life is unlikely
- when considering marriage or other partnerships
- when considering parenthood

of inhalation devices such as ventilators, supplemental oxygen use, etc.

Once the initial introduction and review are completed, and the staff and new patient have developed a rapport, it will be time to discuss the long-term outlook, keeping in mind that CF continues to be a life-shortening illness and that only 50 percent of all people with CF survive to age thirty-six.

All health-care providers are concerned about how well their patients follow treatment instructions, and adolescents are notorious for not always following orders. Patients in this age group with chronic illnesses miss more appointments and more treatments of all types than those in any other age group. Since adolescents normally question all authority, as part of forming their own concept of self in their search for independence, they may be somewhat uncooperative (particularly with medical management) and, at the same time, try to set their own rules for managing their illness. While occasional deviations from treatment are probably not harmful, caregivers have to stress that their patients must accept the treatments as outlined by the CF care team. Compliance is crucial to good CF care, however difficult it may appear for the young person and/or family members.

How Can Parents Promote Cooperation?

Start early—remember that good habits are learned very early in life.

How parents can help

- Provide simple explanations for all questions asked.
- Encourage your child to ask questions about the disease.
- Don't hide information about the diagnosis, treatment or outlook for the illness.
- Provide unconditional love and support at all times.
- Set reasonable goals or rules for diet, medications and physiotherapy.
- Remain consistent in all approaches to the illness.
- Provide the intellectual freedom for your child to develop his or her own ideas and opinions.
- Avoid overprotection.

Encourage independence—never do for children or adolescents what they can do for themselves.

Seek counseling help when the child doesn't want to comply. Both the pediatric and the adult-care teams have counseling resources available.

Promote self-care whenever possible, and always give positive feedback for a job well done or a treatment well taken.

End-of-Life Issues

Although the life expectancy of people with CF has increased dramatically in recent years, cystic fibrosis remains a life-shortening illness. Despite the recent advances in care strategies, such as improved antibiotics to treat infections, better methods and types of nutritional support, new inhaled agents such as DNase, and lung transplantation, we still can't expect a person with CF today to have a normal life expectancy—although we can hope that, with advances in such areas as gene therapy, this will change in the near future. A time will come, for today's CF population, when it will seem unlikely that any further conventional treatment will prolong life for any reasonable length of time. At that point in life, levels of care will be reduced or even stopped, to avoid causing unnecessary fatigue, discomfort or distress in this final period. Changing the level or type of therapy doesn't mean that the CF team has given up. It simply means that the team's efforts will be shifted to providing comfort at this very difficult time. The goal of terminal care is always to provide a maximum of comfort, both physical and emotional, while allowing for the chance of improvement. At this point, it will be important to relieve distressing symptoms.

The most distressing symptom will be shortness of breath related to the progressive lung disease. By this stage most people will already be on supplemental home oxygen. This will continue, and the amount of oxygen may be increased, as needed, to help relieve symptoms. At this point, caregivers may try, or at least consider, other measures to relieve the shortness of breath, by using one or more of the following methods of therapy.

Morphine

Very often, doctors prescribe morphine to relieve the symptom of chest discomfort or pain, but it also relieves the sensation of shortness of breath. Morphine is very effective in relieving these symptoms, and it also provides mild sedation for an anxious patient. Although it can be taken orally, on a regular basis, some people take it by subcutaneous infusion, through a small needle in the skin. They may even inhale it through a nebulizer device.

Minor Tranquilizers

Many people become very anxious during this period, as the effort it takes to breathe increases. A minor tranquilizer such as a benzodiazepine will often help relieve this anxiety, and may provide additional comfort.

Mechanical Ventilation

The question of aggressive intensive-care treatment will almost always arise during this final phase of care. Mechanical ventilation requires that the patient be intubated (have a tube inserted through the mouth into the airway) so that a ventilator can control the breathing. This may prolong life for a short while, but it may also add to the person's discomfort. The CF team will always discourage this method of therapy if the lung disease seems to be progressing naturally, and if there's no hope of extending the person's life with reasonable dignity and comfort.

It's very important that family and friends not isolate the person once this phase begins. They should still encourage him or her to do as much as is possible or comfortable, as far as the symptoms permit. Efforts should focus on making the end of life as dignified and as peaceful as possible.

Advanced Care Directive

The CF staff generally encourage patients to provide an advanced care directive, or "living will," to indicate how they want to live their final days. Each document is written to address the specific needs of an individual, but the document will usually address the following issues.

- It will designate the one person who will make final decisions about care should the patient become incapable of doing so, or of communicating these decisions to the health-care team.
- It will specify whether or not to institute extreme resuscitation measures at any time, should the patient's heart or lungs cease to function, and what the limits of such efforts should be.
- It will say whether to carry out final care in the home, the hospital or a palliative care unit or hospice.

Remember that the person with CF may change his or her advanced care directive at any time. These documents are never "cast in stone," and they can be altered if the person's condition improves.

EIGHT

Issues of Respiratory Therapy

A s we saw in Chapter 3, the airways of people with CF become infected with bacteria from a very early age. Respiratory symptoms and illness develop as the bacteria produce active infections and inflammation in the airways, which leads to the production of large amounts of mucus. The mucus in the airways, in turn, obstructs the normal flow of air in and out of the lung. The major goals of respiratory therapy are to remove the secretions produced by the infection through chest physiotherapy, and to control the bacteria through the use of antibiotics. We'll first look at how secretions can be removed from the infected airways.

Airway Clearance Techniques (Chest Physiotherapy)

From the time of first diagnosis, chest physiotherapy (CPT) has been the major therapy for cystic fibrosis, directed at clearing out the airway secretions. Despite the later addition of many other therapies, such as improved antibiotics for pseudomonas treatment, improved bronchodilator therapy and new treatments like inhaled DNase, CPT continues to be the core of therapy for CF. Over the years, people have come up with many types of physiotherapy techniques, but no one type has emerged as clearly the best. Each CF clinic or physiotherapist may have a preferred method, and no one method should be considered to be "right."

Why Do Chest Physiotherapy?

The secretions that accumulate in CF not only obstruct the airways, but also provide an environment in which bacteria can thrive, invade the lung airways and obstruct the airflow, even damaging lung tissues on occasion. If the airways can be cleared of secretions, and kept clear, lung damage will likely be slowed to a large degree, and the person will have a better chance of living longer.

The ultimate goals of physiotherapy go beyond removing secretions from the airways. The overall goals are to:

- mobilize secretions from the lung and remove them from airways
- maintain normal chest movement
- strengthen and maintain the respiratory muscles
- improve exercise tolerance
- improve self-esteem
- improve quality of life

Choosing a Technique: the Initial Assessment

Because infection and inflammation of the airways occur very early, most CF centers recommend that physiotherapy start as soon as a diagnosis of CF is established. Though chest symptoms may still be minimal, the hope is that physiotherapy will slow down the disease, even at this early stage. Recommended methods vary from clinic to clinic and from country to country. Some methods are more suitable for the infant or younger child, so the approach may change, at the discretion of the physiotherapist, as the person grows older and becomes more independent. Initially, more than one adult should be involved, so that it's not always the same person doing the child's physiotherapy. In general, physiotherapy should be done at least twice a day—after getting up in the morning, and before going to bed. Most important, it should be done *regularly*, and not only when the person becomes acutely ill. With an infant or toddler, physiotherapy will likely involve *postural drainage and percussion*. As the child grows, the techniques will probably be modified to allow the child more independence, but they will always involve some form of drainage procedure.

Types of Physiotherapy

Postural Drainage and Percussion (PD and P)

Among North American CF centers, PD and P has long been considered the "gold standard" for chest physiotherapy. The aim of postural drainage is to allow gravity to naturally drain secretions out of the various areas of the lung. The major airway divides into much smaller airways called bronchi. The bronchi lead to each subdivision, or *lobe*, of the lung, and in a normal person there are five major lobes, three in the right lung and two in the left lung. Each of these smaller airways then divides further, to drain even smaller divisions of the lung called *segments*. Up to eleven segments of the lung are believed to benefit from PD and P. Because the airways to these segments are oriented in different directions, the body has to be moved into different positions, and the airways opening to each of these divisions must thus be aimed downward for a period of time, so that gravity will help maximize drainage. The physiotherapist, or a family member trained in helping with this technique, will then sharply tap (*percuss*) the chest in each position for three to five minutes. Percussion, or vibra-

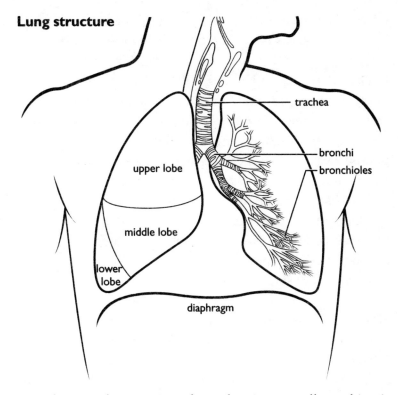

Lung structure

trachea

bronchi

bronchioles

upper lobe

middle lobe

lower lobe

diaphragm

tion, loosens the secretions from the airway walls, making it easier to drain them from the lung. Each lobe, and sometimes even each segment of the lung, can be treated this way, but each has to be treated separately. After one lobe or segment is treated, the person *huffs* (huffing is a special type of cough taught by the physiotherapist) or coughs to expel the loosened secretions that have drained into a larger airway. All this PD and P is best done at least twice a day, preferably early in the morning and just before going to bed.

It's widely accepted that PD and P is beneficial for the continued well-being and long-term survival of someone with CF. Although it's time-consuming both for the person and for any caregiver involved, it should be encouraged for everyone with CF, and is usually started with the onset of symptoms, regardless of the child's age. A major benefit of this technique is that it can be started even with very young children, and it can, of course, be continued right up through adulthood.

Is There Any Reason Not to Do PD and P?

People who suffer from heartburn occasionally find that this form of physiotherapy makes their symptoms worse. With heartburn, acid from the stomach refluxes into the esophagus; putting the person in a head-down position for physiotherapy may increase such drainage from the stomach. There's also a chance that the acid reflux may contribute to lung disease, if the acid refluxes to the point where it can be drawn down into the lungs. Because of this, and because of the discomfort it may produce, PD and P probably shouldn't be done aggressively on anyone who suffers from heartburn.

There's another reason to perhaps avoid this form of therapy. When the posturing requires that the person lie in an essentially head-down position, sometimes the blood oxygen level falls. (This is detected when oxygen saturation measured at the fingertip, by a pulse oximeter, falls during the procedure.) This probably happens because of pressure placed on the diaphragm and the lungs, by the weight of the stomach moving toward the head as the head is lowered. In addition, simply changing the position of the body from upright to a lying position may cause changes in the blood flow in the lungs, which may also contribute to this phenomenon. If the oxygen level falls, probably another technique, that doesn't affect oxygen saturation, should be used.

Despite everyone's good intentions to perform PD and P, it's been shown repeatedly that patient compliance with this technique isn't very good: according to adult studies, as many as 40 percent of people don't follow their physiotherapy program on a regular basis, and don't carry it out to its fullest extent. Because PD and P is very difficult to do anywhere except at home or in a hospital, and is best done with the help of a second person skilled in this technique, physiotherapists and doctors have looked to other methods of providing chest physiotherapy for their patients with CF.

Active Cycle of Breathing Therapy (ACBT)

This is the preferred procedure for physiotherapy in the United Kingdom. It's probably best to delay teaching this technique until the child is at least two years old, simply because he or she has to learn special movements in breathing, and must be able to understand and cooperate with the physiotherapist.

In ACBT, the person is taught a series of steps that emphasize breathing control. He or she starts with normal breathing using only the lower chest and abdominal muscles to produce the breaths, and then gradually increases the volume of each breath, which causes the lung to expand more than usual. As this occurs, the airways open more than they usually would, and air can bypass the secretions in the airway and open any collapsed areas of the lung, so that these can expand and function normally once again. By doing this repeatedly, the person can move the secretions out of the smaller airways. Then, through huffing, the secretions can be moved into the larger airways and expelled out of the lung completely. This is repeated until no sputum is produced for two cycles. ACBT can be combined with postural drainage techniques to remove even more secretions from the lung. Many centers have reported very good results using this method of physiotherapy. Major benefits are that this procedure doesn't require any equipment or a second person to help, and it can be done anywhere—at school, at work or at home.

Because ACBT doesn't seem to decrease the level of blood oxygen, it can be used by people whose oxygen level falls during PD and P. Also, people who have problems with reflux during PD and P can use this technique instead.

Autogenic Drainage

Autogenic drainage means "self-drainage." In this technique, the person breathes in a controlled fashion at three different levels of lung expansion. He or she breathes out almost completely, and then takes several normal-sized breaths at a low level of lung expansion. This loosens mucus from the walls of the small airways. Next, the person allows the lungs to return to a more normal position, and then breathes normally for several breaths. This collects the sticky airway secretions in larger airways. Then the lungs are expanded with a slightly bigger breath, and with the lungs expanded, the person continues breathing in a normal way for several more breaths. This makes the lungs and their airways open up even more, and huffing at this point moves the airway secretions into the major airway, where they can be expelled from the lungs more efficiently.

Autogenic drainage appears to work very well, and some centers feel that it removes sputum better than does PD and P or ACBT. The major problem is that the technique is hard to learn, and it can't easily be taught to children under the age of twelve. However, when correctly used it is very sucessful, and it doesn't appear to aggravate other symptoms such as heartburn. Nor does it seem to cause the blood oxygen level to fall. Another major feature of this technique is that it can be performed anywhere and anytime, and it doesn't require any form of aid or equipment to be effective.

Why Not Just Cough?

When we cough, we tend to close our vocal cords together to block the upper airway, as our lungs become compressed by the respiratory muscles and the chest wall. As our respiratory muscles squeeze the lungs, the vocal cords suddenly open and the air is quickly expelled. Any secretions in the airways are pushed out by the rapidly moving air. Unfortunately, this maneuver also tends to compress the smaller airways within the lungs. When a small airway is already compromised by obstruction or by secretions, coughing may actually make the obstruction worse, so the coughing may prevent secretions from being effectively moved out of the airways. The huffing technique mentioned earlier relies upon keeping the vocal cords open, so that pressures in the airways don't rise dramatically and the airways don't become as compressed as they would be with a cough. Also, coughing causes air to move out of the lungs very quickly, as the vocal cords open, and this rapid movement of air may in itself irritate the airways. This irritation can trigger further spasm, and even block any secretions from being removed from the airway.

Mechanical Aids to Physiotherapy
Several aids have been devised to help clear the airways of secretions. These devices either vibrate the lungs and chest wall, or promote airway clearance by keeping the airways open. None of the following aids has been shown to be better than the methods already outlined. For now, they should be considered only as "add-ons" to the above methods.

PEP Masks
The PEP mask, or *positive expiratory pressure mask*, was developed to hold the airways open during expiration. Every time we breathe out, the natural tendency is for the airways to collapse, and this particularly affects the very small airways in the lungs. This happens even more when we make an effort to cough: the cough increases pressure in the chest, and this pressure is transmitted to the small airways, which forces the airways closed. Keeping the airways slightly open during exhalation might help move secretions out of those very small airways, so a special mask was designed that covers the mouth

and nose. With the mask in place, the person is forced to breathe out through a one-way valve built into the mask. A small resistance in the valve causes the pressure in the airways to increase. Even though the airway pressure increases only very slightly, this means that the airways tend to be held open, and secretions have more room to move out.

Someone using a PEP mask breathes out ten to twenty times, to loosen the airway secretions and allow them to move into the larger airways. Then the huffing maneuver removes the secretions from the airway. This cycle is repeated several times over twenty minutes. The technique is easy to teach, and can even be taught to very young children. Like the active cycle of breathing therapy, this procedure can be done anywhere and at any time; the person only needs to have the PEP mask and valve available.

Oscillating Positive Expiratory Pressure—The Flutter Valve
This device resembles the PEP mask in that it functions by slightly increasing airway pressure during exhalation. It looks something like a pipe, except that in the bowl of the pipe there's a large ball bearing. Breathing out through the pipe stem causes the ball bearing to rise slightly. Because the breathing muscles have to force the air out against the ball bearing, the pressure in the airway rises. The ball bearing then tends to fall back into the bowl, where it plugs the pipe stem until the chest muscles expel enough air to force the ball up again. So, in the course of breathing, the ball rises and falls repeatedly, and this produces a fluctuating pressure, or *flutter*, in the airway. This in turn creates a series of pressure waves that are transmitted backward through the pipe and down into the airways. These pressure waves cause the airway and the mucus to vibrate or flutter, and the secretions become detached from the airway wall. Once the secretions are loosened, they can more easily be expelled from the airways, especially if this technique is

combined with huffing. The procedure is repeated several times, as with the PEP mask.

The flutter valve is a relatively new device and it's still being studied to see how effective it can be, and how it compares with other physiotherapy treatments. It does have the advantage of being very simple—even younger children can easily learn to use it.

Mechanical Percussion and Vibration

Handheld Vibrators

Many people with CF use handheld vibrators to vibrate the chest wall and underlying lung tissue, in conjunction with postural drainage techniques. These devices are designed to substitute for the caregiver who would otherwise provide percussion to the chest wall. The advantage is that the entire PD and P routine can be carried out without the help of another person to do the percussion.

The Vest

This device has only recently been introduced into respiratory care for people with CF. It consists of a sleeveless jacket or vest comprised largely of air-containing pockets. The vest is put on and fitted snugly around the chest with straps. Then it's inflated with air by a special pump. Once inflated, the device rapidly raises and lowers the pressure in the air pockets, and these changes in pressure make the chest wall and the lungs vibrate. This external vibration causes the secretions to come away from the airway walls, and the airways can then be cleared by huffing. A major problem is that the equipment is quite expensive, and probably beyond most people's means. It may find a place in various CF clinics, but its usefulness in the overall physiotherapy picture still isn't certain.

To Exercise or Not to Exercise

The role of exercise in the management of lung disease in CF still remains a bit of a question mark, especially compared to the role of airway clearance techniques. Exercise by itself doesn't appear to affect sputum clearance to any great degree, nor does it seem to benefit lung function significantly. Exercise may improve the clearance of secretions when used along with one of the established airway-clearance techniques.

Exercise does, however, give a sense of well-being and improve self-image. As well, it can improve muscle strength, overall functioning of the heart and lungs, and "exercise tolerance," which is important. With CF, as with CF-related chronic lung disease, respiratory symptoms—in particular, shortness of breath—can make people avoid any physical activity, and this can make their shortness of breath even worse. They end up caught in a vicious cycle that leads to a steady downhill course in their ability to exercise. This decline can be prevented with a structured or supervised exercise program that makes the person feel better psychologically, while maximizing overall physical strength and endurance.

Which Method Should You Use?

Perhaps more important than choosing a method is deciding to *do* the physiotherapy, and to commit to doing it regularly. Physiotherapy has to start with the very earliest symptom or sign of respiratory illness, and many health-care practitioners say that the techniques should be taught even before respiratory symptoms appear. In general, most CF doctors agree that physiotherapy should be started by the time a person produces more than 30cc (about 2 tablespoons) of sputum in one day. With a younger child, it's probably best to use PD and P. As the child grows older, other techniques such as ACBT or autogenic drainage may prove more beneficial. It's usually wisest to decide on a technique in cooperation with the CF physiotherapist, and then review the technique every six to nine months. It's very important that parents of children with CF, other caregivers and physiotherapists commit to working together in this area.

Any of the devices discussed above may prove helpful in physiotherapy, so don't hesitate to discuss them with physiotherapists or the CF doctor, and to try them out.

Antibiotics in CF

As we've noted, the airways of someone with CF will always have bacteria present, and these bacteria will never be completely removed by antibiotics or by any other treatments. However, the use of antibiotics has played a huge role in improving the lifespan of people with CF. This is largely the result of the development of antibiotics effective against pseudomonas, the major bacteria infecting the airways in later childhood and early adulthood. We now have several different antibiotics that are effective against pseudomonas, but most are only available as intravenous medications and don't exist in pill form. Antibiotics are likely to be added to the treatment plan if any of the following conditions is present:

- an increase in the volume of sputum produced on a daily basis
- an increase in cough or shortness of breath
- a decrease in exercise tolerance
- a decrease in appetite or weight
- chills or fevers with no other source of infection
- a drop in oxygen level or an unexplained fall in lung function

Given that those bacteria are always present, and can cause acute, recurring infections, people often ask, Why not take antibiotics on a regular basis to decrease or suppress the growth of these bacteria?

What's a nebulizer?

A nebulizer is a device that forces a constant flow of air to mix with a liquid medication, creating a fine mist which can then be inhaled into the lungs with a normal breath. The process of nebulization requires a compressor device or compressed air tanks attached to the nebulizer to generate the airflow.

This approach has been tried, both with oral antibiotics given daily and, more recently, with nebulization and inhalation of antibiotics, to try to control the growth of the staphylococcus or hemophilus bacteria. However, the people being treated with oral antibiotics didn't appear to benefit over the long term. There's also a major concern with this approach: bacteria may develop a resistance to the drugs, so that when they cause serious infections they'll be much harder to treat. For this reason, long-term administration of oral antibiotics isn't recommended.

Nebulized Antibiotics

During the late 1970s, some doctors and researchers decided to try administering antibiotics by inhalation, a method that studies had shown to work. They reasoned that inhalation could deliver antibiotics to the airways in much higher concentrations than intravenous methods could, so the drugs would be more effective against pseudomonas and other bacteria. This form of treatment seemed to control mild flare-ups of CF-related lung disease, and also yielded modest improvements in pulmonary function tests. However, general interest in using nebulized (aerosol) antibiotics only developed very slowly, and even today the use of inhaled antibiotics varies widely among CF centers. This may change with the introduction of a new preparation of the antibiotic tobramycin, which is gaining attention in the CF community (see below).

Antibiotics that may be administered by nebulizer include:
- colymycin
- tobramycin
- ceftazidime

Of these, colymycin and tobramycin appear to work best. They're now the two most widely and consistently used antibiotics for inhalation.

When to Use Nebulized Antibiotics

Treating Acute but Mild Infections
Respiratory infections or flare-ups in CF tend to recur over time. Unfortunately, everyone with CF can expect to have more than one episode of acute infection involving the lungs. Antibiotics for these infections can be administered orally (only one such antibiotic effective against pseudomonas, ciprofloxacin, is available), by the intravenous route or by a nebulizer. Studies show quite conclusively that treating CF infections with nebulized antibiotics can cure acute flare-ups if they are mild. This treatment won't be used for every flare-up, but it may provide an alternative to using only oral medications, or committing the person to intravenous therapy.

Suppressing Chronic Infections
The use of nebulized antibiotic therapy has recently been studied in people who have been infected primarily by pseudomonas. Most of them had moderate lung disease, with moderate reductions in their PFTs, but they were not acutely ill at the time of treatment. The studies looked specifically at whether lung function could be improved in this group, and whether the use of inhaled antibiotics could decrease the number of admissions to hospital. In the most recent of these studies, patients received

antibiotics for one month and then went off the drugs for the next month; they repeated this cycle several times. Modest increases in PFTs occurred initially, but it's not clear whether this effect will be long-lasting. The studies did show, however, that hospitalizations for flare-ups of CF lung disease decreased among these people.

Can Inhaled Antibiotics Delay Pseudomonas Infections?

The pseudomonas organism, which begins to appear in early childhood, infects people with CF more and more with each passing year. By age eighteen as many as 75 percent have pseudomonas in their sputum. Some CF centers have administered nebulized antibiotics from very early on in childhood, in an attempt to delay the appearance of the pseudomonas. There's still no strong evidence, though, that this approach is working or that it offers future benefits such as extending life expectancy. At present it's not widely accepted as a routine therapy for CF.

What Antibiotics Are Available?

Several antibiotics have been used to treat people with CF, either alone or in combination with a second antibiotic. (When a doctor decides to use intravenous antibiotics, it's standard practice to choose two drugs to which the organism is known to be sensitive. This is done to try to delay or prevent resistance developing to any one antibiotic.) The antibiotics that are most commonly used these days, or appear promising for the future, are described below.

Tobramycin

Tobramycin is very effective against pseudomonas and is one of the most commonly used antibiotics to treat pseudomonas infections. Although introduced as an intravenous antibiotic, it's now widely used for inhalation as well. Most CF centers are familiar with this antibiotic in aerosol form, and are likely to have had good experience with using it for mild flare-ups of lung disease. Recently this antibiotic has been supplied in a form without added preservatives, because there was concern that the preservatives were causing wheezing or shortness of breath in some people.

Tobramycin is administered twice a day by nebulizer. Treatments are carried out for one month, then stopped for a month and restarted for a month, and repeated. Results are encouraging, and treatment with this antibiotic improves PFTs to a modest degree, at least in the short term. This form of treatment has also been shown to reduce the need for intravenous antibiotics, as well as the number of hospitalizations for flareups of CF lung disease. Younger people, particularly those under sixteen years of age, appear to show the best results with this therapy. Older people don't seem to benefit as much, probably because their lung function isn't as good. This therapy hasn't been studied for a very long period of time, as yet, and we don't know whether it will improve long-term survival. Only time will tell if any of its benefits, particularly the improvements in PFTs, can be maintained, or for how long.

Colymycin

Colymycin has proved itself very effective against pseudomonas. It isn't absorbed from the lung into the bloodstream, and therefore it's very safe to inhale it into the airways. Its major benefit appears to be in suppressing pseudomonas infections over a long period of time, although it can also be used to treat sudden but mild flare-ups.

Colymycin hasn't become as popular as tobramycin because it's quite hard to handle. It becomes very sticky when mixed and has a tendency to foam in the nebulizer, making it very difficult to inhale. Occasionally colymycin appears to produce or increase spasm in the airways of the lungs, so that people may complain of wheezing and shortness of breath following a treatment. For these reasons, people tend not to like colymycin as much as tobramycin.

Ceftazidime

This is a very good and potent anti-pseudomonas drug that is mostly used intravenously. It can be used as an aerosol as well, but hasn't proven to be as popular as tobramycin or colymycin for nebulizer therapy.

Intravenous Therapy: at Home or in Hospital

Often a severe flare-up will lead to the decision to start intravenous (IV) antibiotic therapy. Traditionally, this has usually required that the person be admitted to hospital, which allows trained nursing staff to administer the IV antibiotics and maintain the *venous access site*. Because the antibiotics may be administered for up to two or three weeks, a plastic catheter is usually inserted into a vein as an access site, and left in place for the duration of the treatment. A dilute solution of a blood thinner called heparin is put into the catheter between infusions of antibiotics (there may be intervals of three to seven hours when no antibiotic is being infused, depending on which type of antibiotic is used). The heparin prevents blood clots from forming in the tip of the catheter and blocking the catheter. The small amount of heparin used does not affect clotting anywhere else in the body.

There's also ample opportunity in the hospital to make sure the patient gets intensive physiotherapy, and to see that adequate nutrition and body weight are maintained during the period of illness. Increasingly, though, CF centers are embracing the use of home intravenous programs, which show the patient how to self-administer (or show family members how to administer) intravenous antibiotics.

A home IV program is attractive for many reasons, including the following:

- it can be modified to allow people to carry out their daily activities relatively uninterrupted (for example, university students can be treated while on campus and between classes, so that they don't have to miss any of their education)
- it avoids the family disruption of a hospital stay
- it lowers the cost of treatment by reducing the number of hospital admission days

Starting Home IV Therapy for the First Time

People starting home IV therapy for the first time are usually introduced to the process during a hospital stay. This allows the CF team members to teach them how to take care of the apparatus, such as the venous access catheters (the fine tubing that is inserted into the vein—see below), and also the proper handling, mixing, storage and actual administration of the antibiotic chosen. A venous access catheter will be inserted and checked for suitability; it may need to be in place for up to two or three weeks or more, depending on the treatment selected.

Occasionally, staff at an outpatient clinic decide that someone should begin using intravenous antibiotics, for the first time, at home. Most home IV programs are now able to provide first-time setup in an outpatient setting. It may take twenty-four hours to organize all the antibiotics and intravenous equipment, and to teach the patient and family how to do the treatments.

Repeat Treatments of Home IV Therapy

Once the person has been through a course of home IV antibiotics, further treatments may not require admission to hospital. A venous access catheter can often be put in place at the outpatient clinic, and the initial dose of antibiotics can be administered to check for potential drug reactions, and to deal with any concerns the person may have. If the person is very ill, a short hospital admission may be arranged, until the symptoms have been brought under control.

Venous Access Devices

Venous Access Catheter, or Central Line

This long, flexible catheter (tube) is inserted through a needle placed into an arm vein. The catheter is advanced into the vein, and the needle is withdrawn, leaving the catheter in place. The catheter is then advanced 18 to 24 inches (45 to 60 cm) into the vein, until its open tip lies in a large vein in the central part of the chest (hence the term "central line"). The catheter is secured to the arm by tape.

The IV tubing and the IV bag of antibiotics are attached to a closed connector at the outer end of the catheter. When the connector is opened, the antibiotic solution flows into the body. Most antibiotics used to treat CF patients are run in over twenty to thirty minutes, and they are usually administered three to four times per day. When the antibiotic dose is completed, the tubing is flushed with the dilute heparin solution and the connector is closed. The IV tubing and bag may be disconnected for the five to seven hours until the next dose of antibiotics is due, leaving the person free to carry out normal daily activities.

In addition to infusing antibiotics, this system allows blood to be drawn for any blood tests that might be needed. When blood is drawn back through the catheter, the catheter must be flushed with the dilute heparin solution again. The catheters can be left in place for two to three weeks with proper care. Once the treatment is completed, the catheter is simply removed and discarded. With repeated treatments the veins may become scarred or blocked, and it may be necessary to use an *implantable venous access device.*

Implantable Venous Access Devices
These devices are inserted under the skin, by a small surgical procedure. The device consists of two parts: a long plastic catheter, and a self-sealing injection site or "port." The catheter is introduced into a vein and is then connected to the injection port. The port is inserted under the skin, usually on the upper chest or upper abdomen, and the incision is closed over the port, so that there's no permanent opening through the skin. To administer drugs, you place a "gripper"—a small plastic device—on the skin covering the port, and the gripper acts as a guide for a needle to be inserted into the port itself. The IV bag and tubing are then connected to the needle for the administration of the antibiotic.

One advantage of this implanted device is that, once the port and catheter are in place, there's no need to keep re-inserting a catheter into a vein every time antibiotics are started. You can use the injection port up to ten thousand times without worrying about it leaking.

Because the catheter is inserted into a larger vein than is found in the arm, there is much less damage done to this vein, and the larger central veins do not often become blocked. This system may be used either in hospital or at home, whenever IV medications are needed. The only discomfort is the needle prick necessary when the IV needle is inserted into the port itself. Even when they are not in use, the catheter and port must be flushed once a month with dilute heparin solution, to make sure they remain open; this can be done at the outpatient department, or by the patient or family, once they have been taught the proper methods.

Intravenous Antibiotics As Prevention

In North America, intravenous antibiotics are not widely used as a preventive method, to reduce the number or severity of CF lung disease flare-ups. This is largely due to the concern that, as with inhaled antibiotics, bacteria might develop a resistance to the drugs much sooner. Some European cystic fibrosis centers have advocated the use of intravenous antibiotics for prevention, but this necessitates repeated visits to the clinic, or even hospitalizations, and multiple needles for administering the antibiotics. For these reasons the approach has not gained wide acceptance in North American centers.

Inhaled Enzyme Therapy—DNase

When the lungs become infected, white cells from the bloodstream enter the inflamed tissues to try to fight the infection and rid the body of the invading bacteria. As these white blood cells die off, they release DNA protein, which mixes with mucus already in the airways. The combination of DNA and mucus produces the very sticky and thick secretions so familiar to someone with CF.

DNase is an enzyme that can break down DNA. It's normally present in our bodies, where it acts to break down and remove any DNA released from naturally dying white blood cells, or white cells that die while combating infections. It's a normal defense mechanism and we all have it. In people with cystic fibrosis, though, it appears that the naturally produced DNase is overwhelmed by the vast amount of DNA released in the infected lungs.

DNase can be artificially manufactured, and it's available as a liquid that can be nebulized and inhaled. Supplying large amounts of DNase directly to the lungs breaks down the DNA secretion mix, and makes it much thinner and less sticky, so that it's easier to cough up or remove by other methods.

Effects of DNase Treatment

DNase can modestly improve PFTs in people with CF who have moderately severe lung disease. People have also reported additional benefits from DNase therapy, including:

- an increased sense of well-being
- fewer sick days
- fewer days in hospital
- fewer antibiotic treatments
- fewer respiratory symptoms
- fewer lung infections

Is There a Downside to DNase Therapy?

We don't know what effect DNase will have over the long term. The hope is that clearing the airways of secretions will reduce the inflammation and infection, and thus slow down any deterioration in lung function. Everyone with CF, regardless of age, should try DNase, if coughing and, particularly, sputum production are major symptoms. Some CF centers put any CF patient being considered for a lung transplant on DNase until the transplant is carried out, in the hope that the DNase will increase life expectancy, if only by weeks or months, giving the person additional time on the transplant waiting list.

The problem is that this medication is very expensive to use on a daily basis, so third-party payers such as insurance companies tend to resist covering its costs, and will likely continue to do so until we can prove without a doubt that DNase has long-term benefits. Long-term studies are currently underway, and there are also studies looking into the effects of starting DNase in young children, but the results of these studies are not available yet.

Assisted Ventilation

As lung disease progresses with time, the lungs' ability to take up oxygen eventually declines. Low blood levels of oxygen (called *hypoxemia*) can actually make lung function even worse, and thus lower the blood oxygen level even further. To try to slow down this deterioration, doctors may try increasing the blood level of oxygen, which may prolong the person's life to a modest degree. Some form of assisted ventilation may be used:

- to sustain a person who, as the result of a sudden flare-up, suffers acute respiratory failure from a cause that is reversible—for example, acute pneumonia, collapse of a portion of the lung, or a pneumothorax. Once the cause is corrected and blood oxygen levels revert toward normal, the assisted ventilation may be discontinued.

- to sustain a person with chronic respiratory failure who suffers from a natural deterioration or loss of lung tissue and function; in this situation, assisted ventilation will be needed on a day-to-day basis, and probably for the remainder of the person's life.

Supplemental Oxygen

Low blood levels of oxygen can be corrected by providing additional oxygen from a simple oxygen tank, or from a special machine called an *oxygen concentrator*. The concentrator extracts oxygen from the air and delivers it, at a set rate of flow, through plastic tubing and into plastic prongs fitted into the nose. It takes a day or two to get used to wearing the nasal tubing and having oxygen flowing constantly. Occasionally the person complains of a running nose when the oxygen therapy is started, but this lessens over a few days, and is not usually a long-term problem.

When lung disease becomes severe, oxygen levels are very likely to fall at night; even healthy people breathe less deeply at night, and this effect is magnified in people with lung disease. These levels can be monitored by having the person wear the oxygen saturation probe of an oximeter on a finger while sleeping. The oximeter measures the oxygen concentration in the bloodstream and records it with a machine (see Chapter 3 on oximetry). If the oxygen levels fall consistently below 85 percent during sleep, doctors may order supplemental oxygen at night.

As lung disease progresses even further, oxygen levels may continue to fall, to the point where daytime levels are also consistently below 55 mmHg as measured by an arterial blood gas test (remember that a normal level is 80 to 100 mmHg). Once levels get this low, doctors generally recommend that the person use oxygen twenty-four hours a day.

Non-Invasive Positive Pressure Ventilation (NIPPV)

NIPPV is a form of artificial ventilation ("artificial" meaning provided by a machine). It's most likely to be used for very advanced lung disease, where the levels of carbon dioxide in the bloodstream are elevated. NIPPV requires a special ventilator unit that can supply an adjustable amount of air whenever the person breathes in. The air is delivered through tubing connected to a face mask that fits firmly over the nose, and sometimes over the mouth as well. The machine senses when the person breathes in, and supplies an additional amount of air, or a *boost*, through the mask to the lungs. Although this arrangement sounds awkward and uncomfortable, people tend to adjust to it very quickly. Soon they're able to sleep through the night using this apparatus. NIPPV is very good at preventing night-time drops in the oxygen level, but if necessary the machine can supply extra oxygen as well, to make sure the level remains within normal limits during sleep. Most important, these units can prevent the carbon dioxide level from increasing during the night, which is very helpful in preventing morning headaches—often noted when levels of this gas rise at night. People often say they're able to sleep much better and awaken much more refreshed when they use this equipment.

Total Artificial Ventilation

Eventually, and despite all medical therapies, the lungs of people with CF will fail. As this point approaches, it's inevitable that the person and the family will consider prolonging life for days or perhaps weeks through intubation (inserting a tube into the windpipe) and using a ventilator to take over total breathing for the person. This can only be carried out in an intensive care unit, and most centers discourage this form of treatment. While intubation and artificial ventilation may extend life for a short time, this almost never provides either physical or mental comfort for the person being treated, and it should never be undertaken simply for the sake of prolonging life.

NINE

Issues of Eating and Nutrition

The average life expectancy of people with cystic fibrosis has been dramatically increasing over the last twenty years. This improvement has largely occurred for three reasons.

- Several new antibiotics have been developed that are especially effective against the pseudomonas bacteria.
- Improved enzyme preparations have come onto the market, and these are much more effective than the old forms at providing the necessary digestive enzymes that are lost because of pancreatic changes in most people with CF. These enzymes are now used with improved diet strategies, which are tailored to the age of the person and particularly to the unique, changing energy and nutritional demands of each person as he or she grows and matures.
- Early and aggressive care has been introduced in centers or clinics where teams of health professionals specialize in CF care, and where the dietitian plays a key role. Because growth and weight-gain problems start early, contact with a dietitian now begins at the time of diagnosis, and continues regularly through childhood, adolescence and even adulthood when needed. Maintaining good nutrition

ensures that the individual with CF grows normally, main-
tains better pulmonary function and is better able to cope
with flare-ups of the disease.

What Is Malnutrition?

John was transferred to the adult CF clinic with moderately
severe lung disease and a long-standing history of difficulties
keeping his weight up to normal. This weight problem had
been recognized even in early childhood. He'd tried supplemental feedings with a nasogastric tube at night, but he didn't
like passing the tube through his nose every night, and he
couldn't tolerate the sensation of bloating and discomfort that
followed each feeding. Despite a lot of encouragement from
the dietitian and clinic staff, they noted throughout his childhood that he often didn't eat more than 60 percent of his recommended daily calories. After transferring to the adult clinic,
John continued to refuse any form of supplemental feeding,
such as a nasogastric tube or a gastrostomy tube, thinking that
he could always eat enough on his own to keep his weight up.

When he developed a particularly bad lung infection, John
had to be admitted to hospital. During his hospital stay, he
agreed to intravenous feeding, which allowed him to regain
some of his lost weight. After he was discharged, however, his
weight dropped again, and it continued to fall despite encouragement from his dietitian and the clinic staff. As he lost
weight, his cough and shortness of breath also got worse.
Finally, when his dietitian showed him that he was now sev-
enteen pounds lighter than his best-ever weight, John reluc-
tantly agreed to have a gastrostomy tube inserted into his
stomach for supplemental feeding. After a short hospital stay
to have the tube inserted, his dietitian set up a supplemental
feeding program that was delivered by a pump during the
night. Within two months of starting the feeding, John had

regained thirteen pounds, and he had experienced no problems with the gastrostomy tube or the feeding schedule. His lung function also improved and, now that he had a better sense of well-being, he was able to increase all his daily activities.

Adequate nutrition depends on eating a well-balanced diet and having a normally functioning digestive system to break down and absorb the foods we consume each day. As we saw in Chapter 4, the process of digestion involves breaking foods down into particles that can be readily absorbed by the small intestine. These small particles, which may be fats, proteins or carbohydrates, are then delivered via the bloodstream to cells all over the body, which use these substances to produce energy for cell functions, or to create new cells for either body growth or weight gain. Along with the fats, proteins and carbohydrates the body also absorbs numerous vitamins and minerals that it needs. When we don't eat, digest or absorb adequate amounts of any of these substances, growth may slow down and body function may decline. This is called malnutrition.

Why Does Malnutrition Develop?
Malnutrition can develop in three basic ways:
- through increased energy losses
- through decreased energy intake
- through increased energy expenditure

Any or all of these can contribute to malnutrition in a person with CF, and malnutrition can develop at any age.

Increased Energy Losses
By far the greatest energy losses are due to maldigestion and malabsorption of fats and protein, because of pancreatic insufficiency. As we saw in Chapter 4, the majority of people with

CF don't produce enough pancreatic enzymes to adequately digest food, so fats and protein aren't properly absorbed. The end result is poor growth and poor body function. In addition, abnormally thick secretions lining the small intestines may act as a physical barrier, preventing efficient absorption of fats and proteins that have been properly digested. Also, some people have reduced bile acid production and excretion. Bile acids, secreted by the liver, are necessary for the absorption of fats, and of many vital nutrients as well. Finally, people with CF who develop diabetes may suffer from diabetes-related malnutrition (see later in this chapter).

Decreased Energy Intake
A reduction in total energy (calorie) intake can happen for a variety of reasons. Studies show that, for regular daily activities, a person with CF may need 25 to 50 percent more calories than a normal individual. A diet that is healthy for other family members is therefore likely to be inadequate for someone with CF. Diets designed for people with CF contain more dietary fat than normal, in order to provide more calories.

Many medical problems associated with CF can contribute to a reduction in total calorie intake. For example, in the course of an acute lung infection, someone's appetite, not surprisingly, will go down, and he or she may lose a fair amount of weight before the infection is brought under control. As lung disease worsens over time, and lung symptoms become more chronic, people may experience a corresponding loss of appetite for all foods. As symptoms of coughing and shortness of breath increase, appetite decreases; weight is lost and may not readily be gained back.

Depression, a common feature of all chronic illnesses, also affects people with CF. People who become depressed often don't feel like eating, and they may lose weight as a result. Some people even try to lose weight intentionally, in response to current social pressures to be thin. As they try to conform to these pressures, they may actually become malnourished.

Heartburn, as we saw, is a common symptom in people with CF, and involves the reflux of acidic stomach contents into the esophagus. In infants or younger children, severe reflux may lead to vomiting of meals, so they don't absorb enough calories and they may fail to gain weight and grow normally. Severe pain from reflux sometimes causes adults to eat less, in an attempt to avoid heartburn, and these people too lose weight.

Once you become malnourished, it's very hard to gain back the weight you have lost. Even when you are feeling your best, it's often difficult to maintain a calorie intake 30 percent higher than a normal person's, so adding any additional energy to replace lost weight becomes a formidable task. The volumes of food needed may simply be too great for most people with CF to consume through regular eating.

Increased Energy Expenditure

Normal day-to-day activities appear to require people with CF to use more energy than other people do. This seems to be caused by the CF itself, and may be related to the way their body cells process nutrients like dietary sugar and fat. In addition, the progression of CF disease, particularly in the lungs, makes the body consume more energy; more work is being done by the muscles of the chest wall as they move air in and out of the obstructed airways, and in coughing as well.

Deficiencies in Vitamins and Essential Nutrients

Vitamins

The pancreas must function normally for the body to digest fat, as we've seen. But several essential vitamins—vitamins A,

D, E and K—are fat-soluble, meaning that the body can only absorb them from food that contains properly digested fat. We can measure the level of these vitamins in the bloodstream. Even when levels are low, it's rare for this to affect body function right away. However, over time the body may run seriously short of these vitamins, resulting in changes in body functions. (Vitamins that don't depend on fat for absorption, such as the B-complex vitamins and vitamin C, are easy for the body to get from a proper diet, so it seldom runs short of these vitamins.)

Vitamin A

Vitamin A is necessary to maintain normal vision and the normal growth of cells. This vitamin is in foods such as liver, milk, kidney, leafy green vegetables, egg yolk, and yellow-colored fruits and vegetables such as carrots and cantaloupe. When the body runs short of vitamin A, one of the first things that happens is that it's harder to see at night; this is called *night blindness*. When vitamin A deficiency becomes very severe, sores develop on the surfaces of the eyes; if this progresses it can actually lead to blindness. Fortunately, vitamin A deficiency isn't very common, and taking the normal daily requirement of vitamin A will prevent problems.

Vitamin E

Vitamin E turns up in virtually all food groups. It's found in very high levels in such fats as soybean oil, corn oil, sunflower oil and fish oils.

Fortunately, the body doesn't run short of this vitamin very frequently. When there is a shortage, it seems to affect the nervous system most, leading to difficulty in walking or problems with vision. Vitamin E deficiency may also produce anemia in infants. With treatment, symptoms of nervous system disease and anemia generally clear up very quickly.

Vitamin K

This vitamin is found in many vegetable products, and particularly in green vegetables. Vitamin K is essential for normal clotting of the blood. A shortage of vitamin K is most likely to cause problems in infants, where it produces easy bruising. We can solve bruising or clotting problems by adding vitamin K to the diet.

Vitamin D

Vitamin D is actually a hormone produced naturally by the body. The most common source of vitamin D is the ultraviolet light in sunshine, which acts directly on the skin. Vitamin D is responsible for normal calcium metabolism in the body, which we need to produce bone tissue and keep it strong. Shortages of vitamin D in childhood can lead to the development of *rickets*, or very soft bones, which can cause deformities in the growth of bones, particularly in the legs. Adults who don't get enough vitamin D may suffer from *osteopenia*, which literally means "soft bones." When the bone structure becomes severely deprived of calcium, its strength may weaken further and osteoporosis may result, causing bones to fracture easily from even very slight impact. Deficiencies usually occur over long periods of time, so when treatment is necessary it will take a long time too. To ensure that the body receives adequate amounts of vitamin D, particularly during winter months, people with CF take oral vitamin D supplements.

Preventing Vitamin Deficiencies

The best way to deal with vitamin deficiencies is to prevent them in the first place. With good nutrition that allows for adequate fat absorption, the body usually gets enough of vitamins such as A, D, E and K. Since pancreatic enzymes aid fat absorption, it is important for people with CF to take them regularly and in adequate doses. To ensure that the body absorbs enough vitamins, it's a good idea to take supplements of vitamins A, D, E and K. Multivitamin products are available in liquid, children's and adult forms. Specific deficiencies can be corrected by using individual vitamin products, in the recommended number of international units (iu):

- vitamin A: 5,000 to 10,000 iu per day
- vitamin D: 400 to 800 iu per day
- vitamin E: 200 to 400 iu per day
- vitamin K: 2 mg per day

The most common source is a multivitamin including all four vitamins A, D, E and K. Any multivitamin that provides the recommended daily dose of all of the above vitamins will work.

Other Dietary Nutrients—Trace Elements

Iron
A lack of iron results in the development of anemia, or low hemoglobin. Since hemoglobin carries oxygen in the bloodstream to the muscles, people with anemia tend to feel tired and short of breath after very little exertion. This is most common in people who are extremely malnourished or who have severe lung disease. However, it may develop in anyone at any age, and should be routinely looked for on clinic visits. A simple blood test that measures the amount of hemoglobin and the level of iron in the bloodstream reveals its presence. Oral supplements of iron can easily correct the problem.

Calcium
Calcium deficiency probably occurs very commonly in people with CF. Scientists have suspected this since they discovered that people with CF often develop soft bones at an early age.

(See Chapter 6, the section on Osteoporosis.) Treating calcium deficiency usually involves taking calcium tablets, generally combined with oral vitamin D preparations.

Magnesium

Magnesium deficiency is uncommon. However, a few people develop it after taking one of the aminoglycoside group of antibiotics commonly used to treat pseudomonas infections—for example, tobramycin or gentamicin. Symptoms of magnesium deficiency include muscle weakness, muscle cramps and shaking. The symptoms disappear with the use of intravenous magnesium sulfate.

Zinc

Although zinc levels may be low in malnourished people, improving their nutrition will usually improve their zinc stores.

Selenium

Some researchers believe that selenium is part of the normal defense mechanisms against infection within the lungs, but they have not yet found proof, so doctors don't recommend selenium supplements at this time.

Various forms of alternative therapy promote numerous herbal remedies that contain trace metals such as zinc, magnesium and selenium. There is no conclusive evidence to suggest that supplements of any trace metals other than calcium or iron are of any benefit whatsoever in the day-to-day treatment of people with CF, or in their nutritional plans.

Essential Fatty Acids

If the pancreas is not working properly, this will reduce the absorption of linoleic and linolenic acid. Deficiencies of these essential fatty acids are most likely to occur in people with

> ## Measurements monitored to detect malnutrition
>
> Infants, children
> - weight gain
> - height or length
> - head circumference (brain growth)
>
> Children, adolescents
> - weight
> - height
>
> Adolescents, adults
> - weight loss
> - skin-fold thickness (for body fat)
> - arm circumference (for muscle mass)

CF very early in infancy or childhood, usually before the diagnosis of CF. Children with this deficiency have a scaling skin rash and growth failure. They often get infections or bruise easily because they have low levels of platelets (necessary for normal blood clotting) in their bloodstream. When older children and adolescents receive enzyme replacement, it's rare to see them develop essential fatty acid deficiencies. Adding fatty acids to the diet (in the form of corn oil or safflower oil) and ensuring adequate pancreatic enzyme replacement will correct the deficiencies.

How Does Malnutrition Show Up?

Signs of malnutrition may appear at any time from infancy into adulthood. For this reason, both pediatric and adult CF clinics always look for malnutrition. Doctors suspect malnutrition when they see:

- a failure to thrive (in infants)
- a failure to gain expected weight
- a failure to achieve normal growth (height)
- excessive weight loss (usually in adults)

Ideal body weight and nutritional status	
Nutritional status	Percentage of IBW
normal	90–110%
mild malnutrition	80–89%
moderate malnutrition	75–79%
severe malnutrition	below 75%

Dietitians and physicians may describe the severity of malnutrition as mild, moderate or severe. They compare the weight of their patient to the weight of an ideal healthy person, taking into account the height, age and sex of the patient—the *ideal body weight* (IBW). The patient's weight as a percentage of the IBW determines the degree of malnutrition. Infants and young children are monitored with growth charts.

Instituting Nutritional Care Programs
As soon as children are diagnosed with CF, they start a life-long program of nutritional care and follow-up. The aims of this therapy are:

- to optimize growth
- to maintain normal body form and function
- to promote a sense of continued well-being
- to increase life expectancy
- to maintain good exercise capacity
- to promote optimal lung function at all times

Normal nutrition and growth are possible for all children with CF, if parents pay close attention to their individual energy needs and nutritional status.

Nutritional requirements vary for different age groups. Newborn infants and young children need high levels of fat in their diet to meet the needs of their rapid growth. This is the time when enzyme treatment usually begins, since 85 percent of CF infants have an abnormally functioning pancreas and will not be able to produce enough enzymes to carry out normal digestion. Although enzymes do not completely stop malabsorption, enough digestion and absorption of food will occur to allow for normal growth and weight gain.

Where Do Enzymes Come From?

Most enzyme preparations today are extracted from pork pancreas. Because the enzymes are natural biological products, they have a certain shelf life and must always be used before the expiry date. High temperatures, high humidity and exposure to sunlight all limit the effective lifespan of the enzymes, so it's important to protect them from these extremes.

What Types Are Available?

Different types of enzyme products are available but they are all very similar. The enzymes come as loose powder, as powder in gelatin capsules, or as tiny balls or tablets of powder covered with an acid-resistant coating (enteric-coated microspheres— ECM—or microtablets) and taken in gelatin capsules. Enzymes in powdered form may be used for infants, who can't be expected to swallow capsules. It's also possible to open the gelatin capsules and mix the microspheres with applesauce, for even the youngest infant. ECM are resistant to acid secreted by the stomach, and pass into the intestine, mixed with food, unchanged by stomach acids. Once in the intestine, the acid is neutralized by secretions from the intestines, allowing the microspheres of enzyme to dissolve and aid in digestion. Thus ECM are much more effective and efficient in helping digestion than plain, powdered enzyme preparations.

See the chart on enzyme replacement therapy for examples of the usual recommended dose for different age groups, for the enzymes available today.

Enzyme replacement therapy

Age	Food source	Dose of enzyme
Under 12 months	breast-feeding formula	1/2 to 1 capsule per feeding
1–4 years	meals	2 to 3 capsules per meal
	snacks	1 to 2 capsules per snack
5–12 years	meals	3 to 5 capsules per meal
	snacks	1 to 3 capsules per snack
Over 12 years	meals	4 to 6 capsules per meal
	snacks	2 to 3 capsules per snack

ECM = enteric-coated microspheres, 8,000 units of lipase per capsule

Enzymes from different manufacturers may vary slightly in their activity. The effect of different products may seem to vary from lot to lot, and even from purchase to purchase. *Note: to prevent fibrosing colonopathy, do not exceed 10,000 units per kg per day.*

Starting Enzyme Therapy

Once enzyme therapy starts, children should take the enzymes with each meal and with each high-fat snack (it's safe to skip them occasionally if snacks have no fat). Enzymes must be present with the food in the stomach and duodenum for proper digestion. It's usually best to take the enzymes at the beginning of a meal or snack, to ensure good mixing of food and enzyme. Some people have better digestion when they take half the enzyme at the beginning and the remaining half midway through the meal, or even at the end.

How Much Enzyme Should be Taken with Each Meal?

People vary in their requirements for enzymes, and the variation from one person to another may be quite significant. They need to establish for themselves exactly what enzyme product and what strength or amount suits them best. The reasons for

Guide to enzyme use	Meals	Snacks
Starting dose	200 lipase units/lb	100 lipase units/lb
	500 lipase units/kg	250 lipase units/kg
Maximum dose	1,000 lipase units/lb	600 lipase units/lb
	2,500 lipase units/kg	1,250 lipase units/kg

this variation are not entirely clear, but a rough guide to enzyme use for someone over the age of four might look something like the chart in the box.

Obviously, there can be a wide variation in the amount of enzyme any individual person needs. Note, however, that there is a recommended maximum dose. This is to prevent the complication of fibrosing colonopathy thought to be associated with very high lipase enzyme use, discussed in Chapter 4. Increase enzymes slowly from the recommended starting dose, until the child has only one or two well-formed bowel movements per day.

Side Effects of Enzyme Use

Enzymes themselves may cause symptoms. Consuming too much enzyme may result in large amounts of it being passed in the stool, which can lead to irritation of the skin around the rectum and rectal pain. Rarely, children have allergic reactions to the enzymes, which may cause pain in the abdomen and diarrhea. As noted above, excessive amounts of lipase sometimes contribute to the development of fibrosing colonopathy.

Evaluating Nutrition and Growth

Like all other CF therapies, adequate nutrition is a lifelong commitment for the person with CF, the family and the health-care team. From the time of diagnosis, everyone will keep an eye on that nutritional status. There are several ways to rate nutritional status, and no one test can give a true assessment.

Most are indirect methods, beginning with a careful review of the person's dietary history. After this, probably the most useful and reliable indexes of nutritional status are weight and height, as well as variations of these two markers, like skin-fold thickness and upper arm circumference.

Fat Droplet Test
A relatively easy way to judge whether adequate digestion is occurring is to look for partially digested fat droplets in the stools. Unfortunately this isn't always reliable, as the fat content in the diet may vary widely from day to day, so it's necessary to review a positive test carefully.

Fat Balance Studies
Very soon after a CF diagnosis, doctors will want to estimate the total fat content of the stool. They do this by collecting stools from the patient for seventy-two hours and analyzing the amount of fat in them. If the fat content of the stool is more than 7 percent of the digested fat, the gastrointestinal system isn't digesting and absorbing fat properly. This analysis provides the dietitian and the CF doctor with an understanding of how severe the problem is. It may also be used to help them judge how effective enzyme therapy is, and to suggest any changes that might be necessary to provide for good nutrition. This test may be done periodically over the years, to ensure that the person is getting adequate nutrition. It's particularly important to retest people who have poor weight gain, or who have difficulty in maintaining their weight despite adequate enzyme replacement and diet.

Height and Weight
Doctors will keep careful track of the weight and height of a child who has been diagnosed with CF. They'll record both

these measurements in a growth chart, and compare them to the normal growth expected for each month of age. Weight closely reflects the effects of malnutrition, and will indicate its onset very quickly, if it arises.

Skin-fold Thickness

This simple test measures the thickness of a fold of skin held between the arms of a caliper device. The test provides an estimate of the amount of fat stored in the body. Low estimates indicate that the body has not stored fat, or is using it as an energy source. A loss of thickness in the skin fold usually indicates some degree of malnutrition.

Upper Arm Circumference

Measuring the circumference of the upper arm gives an estimate of body muscle mass. If the circumference is less than expected, or less than it used to be, this usually indicates some degree of malnutrition.

Special Considerations in Nutrition

Pregnancy

A pregnant CF mother and her child are both at risk if the mother
- is below her ideal body weight before the pregnancy; **and/or**
- doesn't maintain a normal or expected weight gain during the pregnancy.

Because overall body metabolism increases with pregnancy, a pregnant woman with CF may fail to gain weight, or she may even lose weight, if she's not careful. If you're a woman with CF and you are considering pregnancy, you should try very hard, *before* getting pregnant, to review your nutritional status with an experienced dietitian. Ideally, you should be within 90 percent of your recommended body weight, and you should gain an additional twenty-two to twenty-six pounds (ten to twelve kilos) with the pregnancy. You may need to supplement your diet to achieve these goals, and if you can't gain enough weight with oral supplements, you may need some other form of supplemental feeding—such as a nasogastric tube (see below) for overnight feeding of liquid fat, protein and carbohydrate supplements.

Breast-feeding

Breast-feeding may require an additional calorie intake of 20 percent to maintain normal nutrition in the CF mother. It's certainly to be encouraged, if the mother can maintain a good nutritional status; but if this isn't possible, breast-feeding is not a wise move.

Breast milk from a CF mother is entirely normal. On the plus side, it's better absorbed than infant formula and contains a natural lipase that helps with fat digestion. Breast milk also contains antibodies, which provide natural protection against infections. Remember that if the infant has been diagnosed as having CF as well, he or she will still need enzyme replacement before each breast-feeding.

Diabetes

At present, 15 percent of people with CF develop CF-related diabetes. As we saw in Chapter 4, low insulin levels result in sugar (glucose) levels rising, as the body's cells are unable to metabolize sugar. When the blood sugar reaches a very high level and the kidneys filter it out, into the urine, this valuable source of calories is lost. The body may actually draw on other body tissues, such as fat or muscle, as energy sources. The combination of these two factors causes a loss of body weight, or malnutrition. Insulin replacement therapy will correct these problems and restore normal nutrition. Remember that once insulin is started, it becomes a lifelong treatment with one or more daily injections.

Guidelines for Treatment of Diabetes in CF

- Treat the CF along with the diabetes.
- Provide one-and-a-half times normal energy requirements in the following proportions: 40 percent fat, 20 percent protein, 40 percent carbohydrates.
- Adjust the insulin regimen to the diet.
- Don't attempt to alter the diet to control blood sugar levels.
- Eat three balanced meals and three snacks, spaced evenly throughout the day.
- Include a balance of protein, fat and carbohydrates at every meal.
- Adjust the diet to the individual's needs and be prepared to make compromises.
- Encourage people to participate in self-care programs such as diabetic education clinics, to enable them to adjust their diet and insulin doses themselves.

Adolescence and Early Adulthood

Adolescents, especially girls, may deliberately eat less or decrease their enzyme use to lose weight as they try to achieve the "thin is beautiful" look so fashionable these days, and so important to this age group. The danger is that these young women will lose muscle size and strength as well as weight. This is often reflected in decreasing lung function during this period, because of loss of strength in the muscles used for breathing. Luckily, these losses can usually be reversed once the young person is persuaded to eat properly again.

Nutritional Support and Supplementation

The guidance and expertise provided by a dietitian are a very important part of the nutritional care of someone with CF. Although guidelines for nutritional evaluation and care of the CF patient are now fairly standardized, and agreed upon by most CF clinics in developed countries, it is sometimes necessary to modify these guidelines to suit an individual's needs. Changes may be required because of age group, or the sex of the patient, or to treat specific complications of CF, which can of course vary from person to person. Different methods of dietary supplementation are now available, and most can be adapted for use in any group of patients.

Keep in mind that eating regular foods in the normal manner is, and always will be, the absolute best and preferred way for someone with CF to be nourished. No supplement has been invented that's either better or more natural than simply eating a regular diet. We've seen, though, that the diet of a person with CF should contain 30 to 50 percent more calories than that of a normal person, so diets may need to be modified to provide those extra calories. There are three levels of oral nutritional support available that provide increasing levels of calories:

- level 1—normal oral intake
- level 2—boosted oral nutrition
- level 3—interventional (tube feeding) support

Normal Oral Intake: the High Energy Diet

Since even normal daily growth and activity requirements for the person with CF are 30 to 50 percent higher than for other people, it's recommended, and generally accepted in CF clinics, that the CF diet should contain high fat, for energy production. Very often, it's possible to reach this level by eating regular foods that are high in fat content. If these don't seem to provide enough calories to maintain normal growth and weight, it may be necessary to move to the next step, what is referred to as a *boosted diet.*

Boosted Diet

This is simply a diet in which substances with a higher fat content are added to regular foods. Some ways to do this include:

- using whole milk with 4 percent fat content instead of 1 percent or 2 percent milk
- adding one to two tablespoons of whole cream to breakfast cereal, mashed potatoes or even cream soups
- adding margarine or butter to all vegetables, pasta and sandwiches
- using butter or margarine on all hot foods such as casseroles, cooked cereals, etc.
- spreading cream cheese, peanut butter, honey or jam on all toast, bagels, muffins, pancakes and waffles
- using cream soups rather than broth-based soups
- adding yogurt or sour cream to vegetables, dips, sauces and salad dressings
- preparing instant foods such as cereals, cocoa, puddings and soups with milk rather than water
- having two or three snacks of high-calorie foods between meals, using nuts, milkshakes, pizza or peanut butter to provide additional fat and calories

When a normal or even a boosted diet fails to maintain body weight or growth, it may be necessary to add nutritional supplements to the diet. These can be taken in the form of commercially prepared liquid. Many different kinds are available, and they come in a variety of flavors. People find some more palatable than others, and brand preference appears to be a very individual matter. These products, though, should *never* be used as a substitute for normal foods. They must always be considered as *supplements* to regular meals.

When Feeding Fails—Interventional Support
If weight and height fall below 85 percent of what is expected, despite strong efforts to maintain these with the dietary steps outlined above, some form of interventional support may be recommended. Interventional support usually means introducing a liquid high-calorie food source or supplement directly into either the stomach or the small intestine (jejunum), through some form of tube. Interventional support includes:

- nasogastric tube feeding
- gastrostomy tube feeding
- jejunostomy tube feeding
- parenteral nutrition

Nasogastric Feeding
This involves passing a soft plastic tube through the nose, down the esophagus and into the stomach. The high-calorie liquid food supplement is supplied in a plastic bag, and is usually provided by the dietetic service at the hospital or out-patient clinic. If this service is not available, the person may buy a commercially available food supplement, and put it into a bag. The bag is then connected to the feeding tube and the supplements are slowly pumped directly into the stomach while the person sleeps. At the end of the overnight feeding session, the tube is removed, and it is reinserted before bedtime the next night. The tube is relatively easy to insert, and can easily be inserted by the person with CF.

The person eats normally during the day, and gains a very significant number of calories through the feeding tube at night. After the first few nights, most people have no problem taking liquid supplements this way. While this procedure can be used at home, it may also be used to supplement the calories of people who are very ill and are in hospital.

If nasogastric feeding produces symptoms of nausea or bloating, the procedure can be modified by passing the tube through the stomach and on into the jejunum. Once the tube is in the jejunum, it's left there until the person makes up the nutritional losses, or until the patient is discharged from hospital.

A nasogastric feeding tube

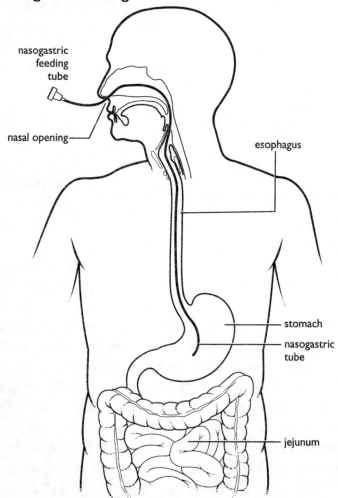

Studies have shown that this system increases growth in younger people with CF, and promotes significant weight gains in all age groups studied. There has been a suggestion, as well, that the use of supplemental feedings slows down deterioration in lung function in all age groups, particularly younger people. The problem has always been to get people to do the supplemental feedings regularly, for prolonged periods of time.

Gastrostomy Tube Feeding

A *percutaneous endoscopic gastrostomy* (PEG) tube is a permanent feeding tube, and is most often used in hospital, when long-term supplement feedings are required. With a permanent tube the person doesn't have to go through the daily inconvenience of inserting the nasogastric tube, or of having a nasogastric or small-bowel tube left in place. This procedure does require minor surgery to put the tube in place. An instrument called a *gastroscope* is passed through the esophagus and down into the stomach. A light on the end of the gastroscope helps the doctor find the best place to insert the feeding tube through the wall of the abdomen and into the stomach. A small connector is then placed in the abdominal wall, leading to the stomach. Feedings are initially started using a connector tube, but subsequently an adapter may be used that allows the feeding tube to be removed. After that, the external feeding tube is attached to the connector for feeding, and removed when no feeding is taking place. This leaves only the small connector, which generally lies very flat on the skin and doesn't interfere with daily activities.

Infusing even small amounts of nutritional supplements into the stomach by either a nasogastric tube or a PEG tube occasionally produces uncomfortable symptoms. Because these supplements are relatively high in fat content, and because they are administered over ten to twelve hours, they add a significant volume of liquid to the stomach. It's not uncommon for people

A percutaneous endoscopic gastrostomy tube (PEG)

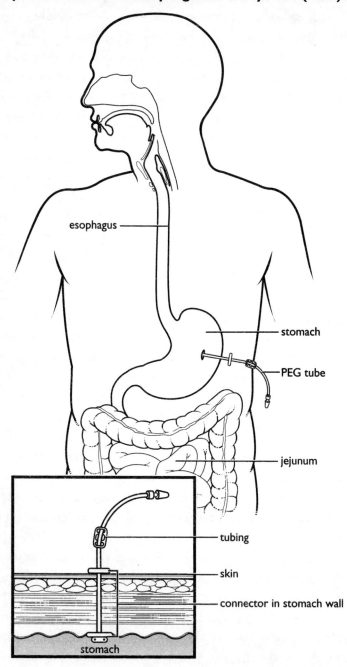

esophagus

stomach

PEG tube

jejunum

tubing

skin

connector in stomach wall

stomach

to complain of bloating; the volume and type of feeding may even produce such nausea that they vomit. As well, if fluids back up into the esophagus, causing reflux from the stomach, heartburn may be so severe that people want to stop this type of feeding. Sometimes medication can be used to make the stomach empty more rapidly, but this doesn't always work, and the person may still want to discontinue the feedings. One solution is to insert the tubing through the surgical opening and advance it through the stomach and into the second section of the small intestine, called the *jejunum*. This method often prevents the symptoms of reflux and heartburn, and it may also lessen the bloating.

Jejunostomy Tube Feeding

Some CF centers suggest inserting the feeding tube directly into the jejunum—a procedure known as a *jejunostomy*. This type of feeding tube is more difficult to insert, so it has to be done under general anesthetic by a surgeon. Standard liquid supplements usually work very well in this situation. Special predigested food supplements are also available, if conventional liquid supplements produce too many symptoms during feedings, such as bloating and diarrhea. This procedure is not commonly done now. Because the PEG tube is much easier to insert, it has become the recommended form of feeding tube.

Parenteral Nutrition

Parenteral nutrition is a short-term form of nutritional support that involves using an infusing pump to get predigested fats, proteins and carbohydrates directly into the bloodstream through an appropriate intravenous site. The liquids are too thick and irritating to be infused into an arm vein, so they have to be put into a larger vein, preferably in the chest. One technique is a PICC line: a central IV line is inserted in the arm vein but it is then advanced until the tip of the catheter reaches one of the major veins in the chest cavity. With proper care, the IV line can be left in place for several weeks at a time. At first, parenteral nutritional supplements are given twenty-four hours a day. Within a week, people usually feel much better and start to put on weight. Eventually the infusion is cut down to twelve hours a day, which provides good nutritional support but allows people more freedom.

A jejunostomy feeding tube

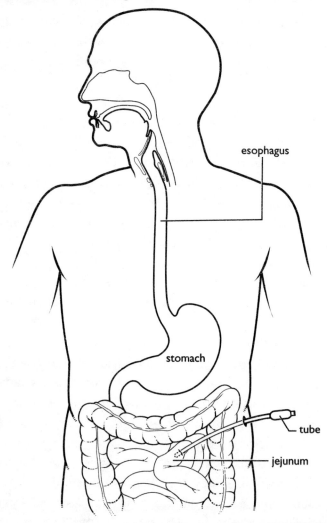

esophagus

stomach

tube

jejunum

> ## Are enzymes necessary for supplemental feedings?
>
> When the usual liquid preparations are used as supplements, they contain substances that need to be digested, just as normal food would be. Therefore, somebody on almost any of the above methods of nutritional support should take additional enzymes at bedtime, to ensure proper digestion and absorption of the nutrients. The exceptions are the specialized predigested diets used with a jejunostomy, which don't require the use of extra enzymes.

Very careful monitoring is necessary with this type of nutritional support. Numerous side effects can occur, because people with CF often have borderline pancreatic function, in terms of insulin production, and the large amounts of carbohydrates they receive through this system can bring on a condition that resembles diabetes. In this case, they may need insulin while they are on parenteral nutrition. Also, the constant high-calorie infusions can cause changes in the liver that resemble hepatitis.

Because of these side effects, and the inconvenience of maintaining the central line and administering the supplements, this form of dietary therapy tends to be used with hospitalized patients only. It's very seldom recommended for use at home.

Short-term Effects of Nutritional Support

When used for short periods such as three to four weeks, nutritional support can have significant benefits. The person may gain a fair amount of weight, experience fewer and less intense symptoms and feel generally better; aspects like lung function may improve measurably. Unfortunately, virtually every CF center that has used this form of nutritional care notes that, once the nutritional support is stopped, all the gains achieved are gradually lost, and people revert to where they were before treatment. Given that periods of supplemental nutrition, via intravenous infusions or feeding tubes, don't produce long-term improvement, it appears that consistently eating a healthy, high-energy diet is the best way for a person with CF to maintain good nutritional health. Parenteral nutrition or feeding tubes should be used when normal nutritional support fails—for example, when the person is acutely ill and in hospital.

Long-term Effects

If providing nutritional support over a period of three to four weeks is not effective, could this kind of support have benefits if used over a longer period of time, such as a year?

Studies show that using parenteral nutrition over longer periods is generally associated with significant problems. Central lines unfortunately tend to be a source of infections, and most people using these lines over the long term need increased amounts of antibiotics to try to control such infections. Sometimes, when an infection can't be controlled, the line has to be changed, causing additional inconvenience for the person. Although people on long-term parenteral nutrition did gain weight, and reported an increased sense of well-being, once the parenteral feeding was stopped they gradually reverted to their pretreatment condition—just like the people who had short-term support.

When Should Supplemental Nutrition Be Used?

Once again, the best method of nutrition for people with CF is *voluntary* eating of high-calorie foods—that is, the person must accept the nutritional plan, and meals must never be confrontational. Only a small number of people will ever be considered for nutritional support, and only when their normal efforts at eating appropriately are not enough or when circumstances such as prolonged or difficult hospitalization require special measures.

Supplemental nutrition may also be considered during certain "risk periods" when malnutrition is more likely—for example:

- when a woman is planning a pregnancy, particularly if she is already malnourished, or is unable to gain weight during a pregnancy
- when a person is significantly underweight prior to serious surgery such as a lung transplant
- during the adolescent growth spurt
- when someone has severe lung disease
- in infancy

TEN

Lung Transplantation and Gene Therapy

In the past fifteen years, great strides have been made in the treatment of CF. One major step is our relatively new ability to transplant human lungs with a reasonable chance of success. However, while short-term results are very good, lung recipients still survive an average of only five to six years after the transplant. In 1989, as the value of lung transplants was being assessed for people with CF who were near death because their lungs were failing, the discovery of the CF gene was reported. This discovery opened the possibility of gene therapy to correct the genetic defect responsible for CF. While lung transplants quickly became common, however, gene therapy has proved to be much more difficult to adapt for clinical use.

Let's first consider the role of lung transplants in CF treatment. The average lifespan for people with CF is now considered to be at least thirty-six to thirty-seven years, and is constantly rising.

The usual cause of death continues to be respiratory failure, which is responsible for 95 percent of all CF-related deaths, and which results from the slow and inevitable destruction of the lungs because of constant obstructions and infections.

Pierre developed respiratory failure from his cystic fibrosis at age twenty-five. Despite aggressive treatment of his lung condition, his lung function had slowly been deteriorating over several years. As his shortness of breath worsened, he found that he had to give up his job as a long-distance truck driver. By the time he was twenty-seven the oxygen in his blood had fallen to very low levels, and he had to go on a home program twenty-four hours a day. At the same time, Pierre was assessed for a lung transplant and went on the waiting list for this procedure.

Within fourteen months, Pierre had an operation to replace both of his lungs. Nine months after the transplant, his lung function was normal and he was allowed to return to his truck-driving job. Now, five years later, he continues to enjoy excellent lung function, and to put in a normal work week, driving his truck all over North America.

A lung transplant is a major undertaking, as it involves extensive surgery and commits the recipient to using immunosuppressant drugs permanently—in addition to all the medications that are needed to treat CF. Since CF affects both lungs, both must be removed and replaced, so that none of the disease-producing bacteria such as pseudomonas remain in the chest cavity. Deciding whether or not to have this operation, and going through the assessment process itself, involve complex and intense decisions for both the person with CF and the family. This chapter will discuss how to conduct this process, and what surgical options are available, and will provide a brief outline of both transplant care and outcomes.

Who Should Be Considered for a Lung Transplant?

Lung transplantation will usually be considered when:

- someone with CF has progressive, severe respiratory failure
- lung function and physical well-being continue to deteriorate despite faithful compliance with medical therapy, physiotherapy and nutritional therapy
- the person has a very poor quality of life and is severely limited in the ability to carry out activities of daily living, **and**
- after due consideration, the person ABSOLUTELY wants to have a lung transplant if possible

There are several aspects of lung function that CF physicians monitor and review regularly to determine when it's time to think about a lung transplant. These include:

- declining pulmonary function test
- rapidly declining pulmonary function test
- deteriorating arterial blood gases
- repeated hospitalization for lung disease

Declining Pulmonary Function Test (PFTs)

Lung function as measured by PFTs is a major method of estimating survival in CF. This is why it's so important to monitor the PFTs on a regular basis. Physicians involved in CF care agree that, once the FEV_1 test falls below 30 percent of normal expected values, the chance of surviving an additional two years is about 50 percent. We also know that the average waiting time for donor lungs is now approaching two years in most centers. For this reason, many doctors feel that they should assess people with CF for a potential lung transplant as soon as FEV_1 falls below 30 percent of its normal, expected value.

Rapidly Declining PFTs

Very occasionally, people with CF experience a much more rapid decline in PFTs than would normally be expected. If CF physicians can't find a cause for this rapid decline, and if intensive medical therapy doesn't help, many centers will assess someone like this for the possibility of a lung transplant.

Arterial Blood Gases (ABG)

Most people with CF are familiar with the discomfort of the needle used for drawing arterial blood gas. This test is very important for many reasons. The levels of oxygen and carbon dioxide in the blood best reflect how well the lungs are functioning. Once the oxygen falls to a level where home oxygen is necessary (see Chapter 3), most doctors will consider the person for a transplant. Similarly, when the carbon dioxide level rises above 45 mmHg, the lungs no longer have any reserve left, and they are failing, so this is also a reason for an assessment for a lung transplant.

Repeated Hospitalizations for Lung Disease

Although this situation is not as clearcut as the indications involving PFTs or ABGs, very frequent admissions for flareups of CF respiratory disease are another reason for considering a lung transplant.

Lung Transplant Procedures

Heart-Lung Transplant

This was the first successful way to transplant lungs. Surgeons transplanted the heart with the lungs connected, in a single block of tissue, after removing the heart and lungs of the person with CF. This is a relatively simple operation technically and produced very good results at first. A major problem was that the recipient had to be placed on a heart-lung bypass machine to maintain blood flow to the brain and the rest of the body. The patient had to receive heparin to thin the blood while on the heart-lung bypass machine, and this sometimes led to significant bleeding after the surgery. In addition, the procedure often damaged the patient's platelets, which are necessary for normal blood clotting. The resulting bleeding in the post-operative recovery room sometimes had to be stopped by a second operation. Over time, other transplant procedures have evolved that don't require use of a heart-lung bypass. As well, the chances for long-term survival are better with these newer procedures.

Bilateral Sequential Lung Transplant

In this procedure, surgeons remove one lung and immediately put a donor lung in its place. Because the new transplanted lung works immediately, they can then remove the remaining diseased lung and put the second donor lung in place without using the heart-lung bypass machine. This is now the favored transplant operation for cystic fibrosis patients.

Living Donor Lobar Transplants

This new approach was recently pioneered by a group of transplant surgeons and physicians in California. Recognizing that more and more people were being added to waiting lists while the number of donors remained the same, they devised a technique to use living donors as the source of new lungs. The surgeons remove a lower lobe of one of the donor's lungs (the small middle lobe is also removed, for technical reasons). Although this constitutes about half the lung, the remaining lobe expands to fill the chest cavity, so the operation actually results in a loss of about 20 percent of the donor's total lung capacity. This does not usually result in any noticeable change in breathing.

The surgeons then transplant that donor lobe into the corresponding side of the CF recipient, after removing the entire diseased lung. Then they repeat the procedure on the other side, using a lobe from a *second* donor. Both donors and recipients do well with this procedure, and the number of these procedures performed has been steadily increasing. A word of caution: because recipients get only about half of each lung, they must be small enough for the lobes to grow to fill all the space within the chest cavity.

At first, only relatives of the CF patients were eligible to donate lobes. Because this procedure has been so successful, most centers now accept non-related donors as well.

When Is a Lung Transplant Not a Good Idea?

As more and more people with CF have successful lung transplants, many fears about potential complications have disappeared. However, any of the following complicating conditions or circumstances may suggest that a transplant is not advisable.

- an acute fungal infection, e.g., aspergillus
- acute tuberculosis
- other organ failure, such as kidney failure or liver failure
- cancer diagnosed within the last five years
- severe malnutrition
- severe osteoporosis
- lack of patient cooperation regarding follow-up or treatment
- testing HIV-positive
- active hepatitis B infection
- prior chemical pleurodesis for pneumothorax
- pseudomonas that resist most antibiotics
- *Burkholderia cepacia*
- an ongoing lifestyle or psychological instability that is likely to interfere with the ability to cope with the surgery, or with taking the necessary drugs regularly after the operation

Aspergillus Infections

This fungus lives in the airway secretions of some people with CF. It usually isn't a serious concern; the organism appears to live happily in the secretions, without causing any significant problems. However, occasionally the fungus gets into a cystic space within the lung, and multiplies, forming a fungal ball or *aspergilloma*. When this happens, there seems to be a very high risk of severe, progressive aspergillus infections in the transplanted lung. Most centers will not perform a transplant when an *aspergilloma* is present in a cystic space. If the fungus shows up only in the lung secretions, the transplant may still go on; the aspergillus is treated with antifungal agents for one month after transplant, and appears to be eradicated by this treatment.

Burkholderia Cepacia Infections

As we saw in Chapter 3, people with CF—and transplant clinics—fear this organism very much, largely because it has resisted most known antibiotics. When transplants first started, this infection would prevent an operation. However, recent experience appears to show that people with cepacia can do as well after surgery as those without it. However, those with cepacia run a higher risk of infections after transplant surgery, and their survival rates are not as good. Some centers perform transplants on people with cepacia; others do not.

Pseudomonas That Resist Most Antibiotics

The situation with pseudomonas that resist most drug treatments is similar to that with cepacia. Given the degree to which the transplant procedure knocks out the recipient's immune system, there is a high risk of untreatable infections with organisms that can resist all antibiotics. Most centers don't accept patients for transplants if they have a pseudomonas bacterium that resists all antibiotics.

Malnutrition

The nutritional status of a possible transplant recipient is extremely important. Most transplant centers won't consider patients whose body weight has fallen below 80 percent of normal, as the outcomes for this group are not as good as for those with normal body weights. Such underweight people would get a transplant only if they first received major efforts to correct any signs of malnutrition.

How Much Does a Lung Transplant Help?

A successful lung transplant is a near miracle to behold. When someone awakens from the anesthetic to say, "My toes are pink," or "I can't feel my breathing any more," it's a marvel and a delight to all of those involved in the transplant. Remember, however, that a lung transplant can't restore a normal life expectancy to a person with CF, nor will it affect any of the other problems associated with the disorder. The recipient will still have to take all the other treatments, such as enzyme and vitamin supplements, and must continually work at maintaining well-being and nutrition. All the same, a successful transplant can significantly improve the length and quality of life.

How Long Will a Transplanted Lung Work?

After a lung transplant, the recipient must take drugs to suppress the immune system from that day on. Rejection remains a constant threat. Ultimately every transplanted organ will be rejected, but because of its delicate nature, the lung appears much more prone to rejection, and strict attention must be paid to suppressing the immune system's reaction to the foreign lung. At the present time, 55 to 60 percent of people with CF who have lung transplants survive for at least five years. Survival rates have been steadily improving as researchers refine and improve immunosuppression medications. We can only hope that these improvements will yield even longer survival times within the foreseeable future.

Can the Cystic Fibrosis Gene Be Fixed?

Once scientists identified the CF gene in 1989, tremendous hope arose that a cure for CF might soon become available. Before long, however, researchers discovered that more than one type of gene defect could be involved, and now we recognize more than 850 different gene defects related to CF. All these defects have one thing in common: they appear to affect the functioning of the CFTR protein, the very small channel in the cell surface lining various duct systems. Researchers hoped that, with modern techniques, they could replace the entire gene. If they could do this, they could treat all the various organs that are damaged by CF. Since we can only detect the disease after birth, when the organs have already formed, gene therapy would have to be aimed at a specific organ, and would only correct the defect within that organ. At present there is still no way to correct the gene defect before birth, when the fetus is just developing. But with so many organs involved in CF, where would we start trying to correct the defects?

The first candidate selected for gene therapy was the lung, for two major reasons. The obvious reason was that lung failure ultimately leads to the death of 95 percent of people with CF, so there is an urgent need for gene therapy in the lungs. The second reason was that whatever genetic material had to be introduced into the lungs could be easily inhaled as an aerosol solution. This genetic material would then specifically target the cells lining the airways in the lungs.

How Can You Change the Genes in Someone's Lungs?

Once the CF gene had been identified, scientists were able to produce a normal human CFTR gene artificially. The next step was to introduce this normal CFTR gene into the cells lining the airways, to try to induce those cells to produce normal CFTR protein. The cells might then be able to produce healthy airway secretions. This in turn might restore the normal defense mechanisms within the airways to prevent further infections and inflammation—which would spare the airways and lung tissue from further destruction.

The normal gene product must not only get inside the cell, it must become *part* of the gene apparatus within the cell. Can this be done? Viruses do something very similar to this all the time. A virus such as influenza gets into a cell and inserts its own genetic material into the genetic machinery of the cell. The virus virtually takes over the functions of that cell; this is how viruses normally reproduce, and how they are able to survive. It is relatively simple for scientists nowadays to introduce CFTR gene material into a virus, and to have the virus "think" this is part of its own genetic material. If we could find a virus that would enter the cell that has the CFTR gene, perhaps the virus would override the defective genetic material; the infected cell would then be able to produce normal CFTR protein.

The virus that was chosen is called the *adenovirus*. The adenovirus was appropriately altered and was then sprayed into the airways of a few volunteers, and allowed to penetrate the airway cells.

In early studies, this was done by inserting a bronchoscope down into a lobe of the lung; a technician then squirted a solution containing the virus down a small channel in the bronchoscope, which allowed it to flow into the various small airways within the lobe of the lung. Although the area within the lung (and hence the number of cells affected) was very small, some genetic material could be inserted to at least partially correct the defect in the CFTR protein. Unfortunately this was a very difficult procedure, because of the discomfort caused by passing the bronchoscope into the lung, and the fact that it could infuse the solution into only very small areas of the lung at any one time. The major benefit of this research, which took many years to accomplish, was to demonstrate that the process did work. The next questions were whether the results would last long, and whether a more effective method could be found.

Unfortunately, in most of the studies done, the airway cells did produce CFTR protein at first but the effects declined over time. This posed a major problem, as it suggested that the procedure would have to be repeated on some regular basis. To overcome this obstacle, researchers have considered the possibility of modifying the virus, or finding some other type of *vector* (carrier) that produces more lasting effects.

Where Are We Now in Gene Therapy?

Despite ten years of gene therapy research, no one has yet found a much more efficient system to introduce correct genetic material into the affected cells. One of the reasons for our limited success with the adenovirus is the body's natural defense mechanism against this virus: the immune system forms antibodies that destroy it. Repeatedly sending this virus into the lungs just means that the body gets better and better at destroying it. Researchers are still looking for other vectors to carry the gene material into the airway cells.

Adeno-associated Viruses (AAV)

These very small viruses can penetrate the airway cells in much the way the adenovirus does. They seem to be better carriers than the adenovirus, but unfortunately, at the present time, it's not possible to develop large enough quantities of such a very small virus for widespread use. Like adenovirus treatment, AAV treatment is still used only for research purposes.

Non-viral Vectors

Scientists are now investigating *non-viral vectors*. A type of normally occurring fat (lipid) that circulates in the bloodstream can carry CFTR genetic material. The airway cells can absorb a combination of the lipid and the genetic material, and add the genetic material to the cell gene structure. Once this occurs, the cell can produce normal CFTR protein. This has turned out to be a very inefficient system, for many reasons, but when it does work it yields normal-appearing CFTR protein. Researchers are continuing to work with lipids in the hope of finding one that lets the cells produce normal CFTR protein more efficiently.

Prospects for the Future

Gene therapy remains a promising approach to the treatment of CF lung disease. Progress has been slow—certainly much slower than anybody anticipated—but we continue to move forward. We hope that one day we will have an efficient vector to penetrate the lung cells and repair them permanently. Eventually, we hope, we will be able to repair the defective genes in all the organs affected by CF.

Cystic fibrosis is a complex disease that does terrible damage to the lives of young people and their families. Many researchers are devoting their lives to finding a way to cure it. Sometime—sooner or later—we will find the answer.

Table of Drug Names

Drug Type	Generic Name	Common Brand Names
Antibiotic	Ceftazidime	Ceptaz, Fortaz, Tazidime
	Ciprofloxacin	Cipro
	Cloxacillin	Cloxapen*, Orbenin†
	Colymycin	Colistin
	Tobramycin	Nebcin, TOBI
Glucocorticoid	Prednisone	Apo-Prednisone
Painkiller	Morphine	MS Contin
Immunosuppressant	Cyclosporine	Neoral, Sandimmune
	Azathioprine	Imuran
Bisphosphonate *(osteoporosis treatment)*	Alendronate	Fosamax
Pancreatic enzyme	Pancrelipase	Cotazym, Pancrease, Viokase
Sedatives *(benzodiazepines)*	Diazepam	Valium
	Lorazepam	Ativan
Sputum liquefier enzyme	DNase	Pulmozyme
Bile salt replacement	Ursodeoxycholic acid	Urso
Laxative	Polyethylene glycol	Colyte, GoLYTELY

†Available in Canada only
*Available in U.S. only

Glossary

Active cycle of breathing therapy (ACBT): a technique used in physiotherapy to promote removal of secretions from the lung.

Addison's disease: the failure of adrenal glands to secrete normal levels of blood hormones such as adrenalin.

Adeno-associated viruses (AAV): viruses very similar to the adenovirus (see below) and also used in gene therapy studies.

Adenovirus: a virus which commonly infects the human respiratory system and pro-duces a cold-like illness; often used in gene therapy studies.

Adrenal insufficiency: failure of the adrenal gland to produce and secrete normal levels of hormones such as adrenalin. Also called Addison's disease.

Amylase: an enzyme that digests carbohydrates.

Arterial blood gas test (ABG): a test to measure levels of oxygen and carbon dioxide in the bloodstream.

Arthralgia: pain or discomfort in a joint.

Assisted ventilation: the use of a mechanical air pump (ventilator) to send air into the lungs.

Atelectasis: the collapse of a portion of the lung, so that no air remains it.

Autogenic drainage: a tech-nique used in physiotherapy to promote drainage of secretions from the airways.

Bile: the liver's main secretion, necessary for normal digestion.

Bile salts: the main chemical in bile.

Bilirubin: a substance created by the breakdown of red blood cells, removed by the liver and secreted in the bile. Bilirubin produces the common orange-green color of bile.

Bronchioles: very small airways in the lungs.

Bronchiolitis: obstruction and inflammation of the bronchioles.

Bronchiectasis: a condition in which damaged bronchioles "balloon" to form cyst-like areas.

Bronchodilators: inhaled medications that widen con-stricted air passages, making breathing easier.

Cepacia: a type of bacterium which can infect the airways in people with cystic fibrosis.

Chest physiotherapy (CPT): various techniques used to promote drainage of secretions from the lungs and promote more efficient breathing.

Cholecystitis: inflammation of the gallbladder.

Chorionic villus sampling: a prenatal procedure to remove cells from the placenta for genetic testing.

Chromosomes: molecules that carry hereditary information. Each human cell contains 23 matched pairs of chromosomes, one of each pair from the mother, the other from the father.

Cilia: hair-like projections on the surface of airway cells that beat continuously to sweep out mucus, bacteria and trapped particles.

Cirrhosis: fibrosis or scarring of the liver.

Clubbing: enlargement and rounding of the ends of fingers and toes.

Computerized tomography (CT) scan: an X-ray technique that produces an image of the brain by computerized assem-bly of X-ray images.

Corticosteroids: medications used to reduce inflammation resulting from infection in the airways; commonly adminis-tered through a small hand-held inhaler, but also available in pill or intravenous forms.

Deoxyribonuclease (DNase): an enzyme that breaks down the protein DNA (see below).

Deoxyribonucleic acid (DNA): the chemical structure of genes, which forms the genetic code determining inherited characteristics.

DEXA scan: a bone scan that measures bone mass (density).

Distal intestinal obstruction syndrome (DIOS): abdominal pain and distension that occur when the end of the small intestine becomes obstructed by thick secretions and food contents.

DNA: *see* **Deoxyribonucleic acid.**

DNase: *see* **Deoxyribonuclease.**

ECM: *see* **Enteric-coated microspheres.**

Enteric-coated microspheres (ECM): small pellets of pancreatic enzymes with an acid-resistant coating; these pass through the stomach and become active in the small intestine.

Enzyme therapy: replacing reduced or absent pancreatic enzymes with enzymes taken by mouth at each meal.

Failure to thrive: malnutrition in infancy.

Fat balance studies: studies determining the amount of dietary fats absorbed by digestion or eliminated in the stool.

Fat droplet test: a test demonstrating the level of fat droplets in the stool.

FEV_1: *see* **Forced expiration volume.**

Fibrosing colonopathy: severe inflammation and scarring in the large bowel, produced by ingesting high doses of pancreatic enzymes.

Flutter valve: *see* **Oscillating positive expiratory pressure.**

Focal biliary fibrosis: small areas of scarring within the liver.

Forced expiration volume (FEV_1): a test that measures the amount of air pushed out of the lungs in the first second of a forceful exhaled breath.

Gastroesophageal reflux disease (GERD): inflammation in the lower esophagus produced by regurgitation of acid from the stomach, commonly causing the pain popularly known as heartburn.

Gastrostomy tube feeding: pumping liquid preparations of basic food nutrients through a feeding tube into the stomach.

Genotyping: tests to detect and identify a specific gene.

Hemoglobin A-1-c: a combination of hemoglobin in red blood cells with blood glucose. Measurement of A-1-c levels in the blood is an indication of whether the body's blood sugar is being adequately controlled.

Hemoptysis: coughing up blood.

Hyperalimentation: increased amounts of nutritional supplements administered through a feeding tube into the stomach or small bowel.

Hypertrophic pulmonary osteoarthropathy (HPOA): a painful condition involving the long bones of the legs and occasionally arms, thought to result from swelling in the covering of the bones, produced by low blood oxygen levels.

Hypoparathyroidism: low or reduced functioning of the parathyroid glands, which control calcium metabolism and bone growth.

Hypothyroidism: a condition which results from decreased production of thyroid hormone by the thyroid gland.

Huffing: a special type of cough taught by a physiotherapist.

Hypoxemia: a low level of oxygen in the bloodstream.

Immunoreactive trypsin test (IRT): a blood test to detect increased pancreatic enzymes in the bloodstream of newborns with cystic fibrosis.

Insulin: a hormone produced by the pancreas that controls the body's absorption of glucose (sugar).

Intubation: inserting a plastic tube into the airway to allow assisted ventilation.

Intussusception: a condition in which the bowel folds into itself, causing a valve-like obstruction.

Jejunostomy: creation of an opening into the jejunum for the purpose of introducing a feeding tube.

Jejunum: the mid-portion of the small intestine.

Laparoscope: a fiberoptic telescope-like instrument which can be inserted into the abdomen to inspect the abdominal organs.

Lipase: an enzyme that digests fats.

Lithotripsy: breaking up kidney stones by focusing ultrasonic waves on them.

Lobar transplant: transplantation of a single lobe of a lung, usually a lower lobe.

Lobe of a lung: the largest subdivision of a lung—an upper, middle or lower lobe of the right lung or the upper or lower lobe of the left lung.

Lobectomy: removal of a single lobe of a lung.

Meconium: a mucous substance present in the intestines at birth.

Meconium ileus: a bowel obstruction caused by very thick meconium.

Meconium ileus equivalent: a type of obstruction within the small bowel (see **Distal intestinal obstruction syndrome**).

Micro gallbladder: a smaller than normal gallbladder.

Multilobular biliary cirrhosis: widespread, often very severe scarring or fibrosis within the liver.

Nasal polyp: localized swelling of the lining of the nasal cavity.

Nasoscope: small telescope-like instrument used to inspect, irrigate and drain the nasal passage.

Nasogastric feeding: supplying supplemental feeding through a tube passed through the nose until its tip is in the stomach.

Nebulizer: a device using a power source and compressor to deliver a mist of aerosolized medication, usually through a mask.

Non-invasive positive pressure ventilation (NIPPV): a form of assisted or artificial ventilation supplied through a face mask covering the nose and mouth.

Oral hypoglycemic agents: medication taken by mouth to lower blood sugar levels.

Oscillating positive expiratory pressure: a pressure wave produced in the airway by blowing through a flutter valve.

Osteopenia: a softening of bones produced by poor formation of bone structure, considered the beginning of osteoporosis.

Osteoporosis: bone disease characterized by reduced bone density.

Oximetry: a measurement of the level of oxygen in the blood.

Oxygen concentrator: a machine that extracts oxygen from the air and delivers it to someone through nasal tubing.

Parenteral feeding: administering nutrients directly into the body through a tube inserted in a vein.

Percutaneous endoscopic gastrostomy (PEG) tube: a feeding tube inserted through the skin of the abdomen into the stomach.

Plasma lipids: digested fats circulating in the bloodstream.

Pleurodesis: a procedure to make the lung adhere to the chest wall, commonly used to treat a pneumothorax.

Pneumothorax: collapse of a lung when air leaks from the lung into the chest cavity.

Polypectomy: surgical removal of polyps.

Portal hypertension: increased pressure in the veins of the abdomen, as a result of cirrhosis.

Positive expiratory pressure (PEP) mask: a face mask used during physiotherapy to create increased pressure in the mouth and airways during exhalation. The pressure helps keep the airway open and promotes drainage of mucus from the lungs.

Postural drainage and percussion (PD and P): a physiotherapy technique that positions the patient to drain mucus from the lung while percussing (repeatedly striking) the chest wall.

Protease: an enzyme that digests protein.

Pseudomonas: a type of bacteria that commonly infects the lungs of people with cystic fibrosis.

Pulmonary function testing (PFT): tests to measure changes in lung function.

Rectal prolapse: a bulging of the lining of the large bowel that protrudes through the rectum.

Sinusitis: sinus swelling and inflammation.

Spirometry: a technique measuring airflow in the lung.

Sweat chloride test: a measure of the chloride ion content of sweat.

Ursodeoxycholic acid (UDCA): a medication used to treat liver changes in people with cystic fibrosis.

Varices: dilated blood vessels in the lower esophagus and stomach; a result of the development of portal hypertension.

Venous access device: a small metal and rubber reservoir used to administer intravenous solutions, usually inserted permanently beneath the skin. The reservoir is connected to a large vein by a small attached tube.

Further Resources

Organizations

U.S.A.

Cystic Fibrosis Foundation
6931 Arlington Road
Bethesda MD   20814
(301) 951-4422
Toll-Free: 1-800-FIGHT CF
    (344-4823)
www.cff.org

American Dietetic Association
216 West Jackson Boulevard
Chicago IL   60606-6995
(312) 899-0040
www.eatright.org

Canada

**Canadian Cystic Fibrosis
    Foundation**
2221 Yonge Street, Suite 601
Toronto ON   M4S 2B4
(416) 485-9149
Toll-Free: 1-800-378-2233
    (Canada only)
www.cysticfibrosis.ca

Dietitians of Canada
480 University Avenue,
    Suite 604
Toronto ON   M5G 1V2
(416) 596-0857
www.dietitians.ca

Other Websites

Cystic Fibrosis Trust Organization, United Kingdom
(Well-organized and detailed information source)
www.cftrust.org.uk

Books

Orenstein, Dr. David, Dr. Beryl Rosenstein and Dr. Robert Stern. *Cystic Fibrosis: Medical Care*. Baltimore: Lippincott William and Wilkins, 2000.

Parker, Dr. J., and Dr. P. Parker. *The 2002 Official Parents' Source Book on Cystic Fibrosis*. San Diego: ICON Health Publications, 2002.

Index

A page number in italic indicates a figure, table or boxed text. For drug brands please see the table of drug names on page 170.